Lourdes M. Cuéllar

Diane B. Ginsburg

D1073618

Preceptor's Handbook for Pharmacists

American Society of Health-System Pharmacists®

Bethesda, Maryland

Any correspondence regarding this publication should be sent to the publisher, American Society of Health-System Pharmacists, 7272 Wisconsin Avenue, Bethesda, MD 20814, attention: Special Publishing.

The information presented herein reflects the opinions of the contributors and advisors. It should not be interpreted as an official policy of ASHP or as an endorsement of any product.

Because of ongoing research and improvements in technology, the information and its applications contained in this text are constantly evolving and are subject to the professional judgment and interpretation of the practitioner due to the uniqueness of a clinical situation. The editors, contributors, and ASHP have made reasonable efforts to ensure the accuracy and appropriateness of the information presented in this document. However, any user of this information is advised that the editors, contributors, advisors, and ASHP are not responsible for the continued currency of the information, for any errors or omissions, and/or for any consequences arising from the use of the information in the document in any and all practice settings. Any reader of this document is cautioned that ASHP makes no representation, guarantee, or warranty, express or implied, as to the accuracy and appropriateness of the information contained in this document and specifically disclaims any liability to any party for the accuracy and/or completeness of the material or for any damages arising out of the use or non-use of any of the information contained in this document.

Director, Special Publishing: Jack Bruggeman
Acquisitions Editor: Rebecca Olson
Developmental Editor: Robyn Alvarez
Senior Editorial Project Manager: Dana Battaglia
Production Editor: Kristin Eckles
Cover Design: DeVall Advertising
Page Design: Armen Kojoyian, David Wade

Library of Congress Cataloging-in-Publication Data

Preceptor's handbook for pharmacists / [edited by] Lourdes M. Cuéllar, Diane B. Ginsburg. — 2nd ed.
     p. ; cm.
  Includes bibliographical references and index.
  ISBN 978-1-58528-203-6
  1. Pharmacy—Study and teaching—United States—Handbooks, manuals, etc. 2. Medicine—Study and teaching (Preceptorship)—United States—Handbooks, manuals, etc. I. Cuéllar, Lourdes M. II. Ginsburg, Diane B. III. American Society of Health-System Pharmacists.
  [DNLM: 1. Education, Pharmacy—methods. 2. Preceptorship—methods. QV 20 P923 2009]
  RS110.P74 2009
  615'.1076—dc22
                                            2009018750

ISBN 978-1-58528-203-6

We dedicate this edition to those who have the passion to give back to others; those who understand the importance of giving. Maya Angelou said it best in the following quote: "I have found that among its other benefits, giving liberates the soul of the giver."

We are especially thankful to those who have given to us throughout our lives, our late parents, Phyllis Ginsburg, and Celso and Matiana Cuéllar. We honor their memories by giving to others.

Table of Contents

CHAPTER 1

   Sara J. White, Kevin Purcell, Randy Ball, Lourdes M. Cuéllar

CHAPTER 2

   Sara J. White, Diane B. Ginsburg, Lee C. Vermeulen,
   Stacy A. Taylor, Michael Piñón

CHAPTER 3

   Dana S. Fitzsimmons, James Colbert, Jr., Roy T. Hendley,
   Grace M. Kuo, Andrew Laegeler, Jennifer L. Ridings-Myhra

CHAPTER 4

   Debra S. Devereaux

CHAPTER 5

   Dale E. English II, Linda Stevens Albrecht, Ruth E. Nemire,
   Traci L. Metting

Acknowledgments

Webster defines *passion* as, "extreme, compelling emotion; intense emotional drive or excitement." When one decides to teach another, it is this emotion, this excitement about seeing others develop that overcomes and satisfies this passion and encourages us to do more. To teach is to have the passion and dedication in others, a true selfless act knowing that others will be the beneficiaries of your time and commitment. This passion is at the very core of what we do as individuals and professionally as practitioners.

When we started the first edition, we knew there were many out there like us who shared this same passion for teaching and developing others. As with the first edition, we have been fortunate to work with so many others who understand this passion in the writing of this handbook. Certainly anyone who has ever precepted a student knows the importance of giving back to the profession by assisting in the development of its future practitioners. We are truly grateful to all who have contributed to this edition and thank you for your commitment to the future of this profession. As with the first edition, we hope this text continues to be a valuable guide for those who are embarking on this aspect of their practice. There are few things more rewarding than knowing and seeing that you have indeed helped develop another.

We want to thank those who have impressed upon us the importance of giving back, the many students we have taught over the years. All of you have taught us many important lessons and are the reason why we both actively teach today. All of you have touched our lives in immeasurable ways, and we are committed to those who will be teaching in the future.

We want to thank our editors and staff at ASHP for their assistance with the publication of the second edition. We are greatly appreciative of your support, insight, and understanding of the need for this type of guide for practitioners.

In addition, we want to thank the true inspirations in our lives, our late parents, who instilled in each of us the importance of giving back and helping others. We were fortunate to have had such incredible role models in our lives. We honor their memory by our giving to others.

Lourdes M. Cuéllar, MS, R.Ph., FASHP
Diane B. Ginsburg, MS, R.Ph., FASHP

Foreword

With the implementation of updated and new standards for accreditation of schools of pharmacy, the Accreditation Council for Pharmacy Education (ACPE) has placed a broader and deeper emphasis on experiential education.[1] These standards require that schools include two types of experiential education in the pharmacy curriculum: introductory experiences and advanced practice experiences. The former are designed to provide the pharmacy student with experiences that allow for introductions to various types of practice in a diverse set of sites. The latter are contemplated to engage the student in problem-solving around therapeutic issues in a variety of areas of specialty practice in both the inpatient and outpatient setting. Taken together, experiential education requirements in the contemporary curriculum represent more than 20% of total curricular time. This places an immense responsibility on preceptors within and outside of the University setting.

To that end, having individual preceptors properly trained for this critical responsibility has become a challenging task for the schools. But were it not for mostly volunteer efforts of preceptors, implementing the experiential curricular requirements would be a significant challenge and burden to the schools. Responsible preceptorship carries with it an active engagement with aspiring professionals to inculcate the values, culture, ethics and patient care centeredness of the profession of pharmacy. It also provides an unparallel opportunity to shape the career goals on students.

But preceptorship does not come totally naturally. It requires patience, dedication, planning, mentorship and role modeling. Training for these roles, in addition to staying current with practice and patient care, becomes an important factor for both the schools and the profession. Moreover, the precepting role must constantly adapt to changes in practice, education and the external environment in which the practice exists. Increasing complexity of drug therapy, coupled with increasing cost pressures for efficiency and efficacy, require preceptors to be studious guides to students under their care.

It will be increasingly important that preceptors not merely transfer their skills to students. That is apprenticeship. Rather, preceptors have a responsibility and professional duty to assure that the experiential component of the curriculum brings to life the class room learnings and patient care implications for assuring rational drug therapy. That requires careful tutoring, strong review and feedback, constant oversight of key concepts in quality and safety as well as personal trait development. That is no small task.

In this edition of Cuellar's and Ginsburg's *Preceptor's Handbook for Pharmacists*, the authors affirm these concepts. By applying the guidance provided in this handbook, practitioner teachers can resist vocationalism and strengthen their abilities to truly precept and mentor students in both application of theory and fact and shaping attitudes and behaviors. This latter point will be increasingly important for the profession; namely, that its aspirants derive meaning from their experiences and that preceptors will be recalled as individuals who have had an impact on the clarification of values and attitudes in the profession. The continuous, constructive evolution of the profession of pharmacy will rely on preceptors having had that type of impact on its new members.

Henri R. Manasse, Jr., Ph.D., Sc.D., FFIP
Executive Vice President and Chief Executive Officer
American Society of Health-System Pharmacists
Professional Secretary
International Pharmaceutical Federation
March, 2009

---

[1] Accreditation Standards, Accreditation Council for Pharmacy Education, 2009, Chicago, IL.

Editors

Lourdes M. Cuéllar, MS, R.Ph., FASHP
Director of Pharmacy & Clinical Support Services
TIRR Memorial Hermann
Adjunct Clinical Professor
University of Houston College of Pharmacy
Houston, Texas
Adjunct Clinical Associate Professor
Feik School of Pharmacy
University of the Incarnate Word
San Antonio, Texas

Diane B. Ginsburg, MS, R.Ph., FASHP
Clinical Professor
Assistant Dean for Student Affairs
Regional Director, Internship Program
College of Pharmacy
The University of Texas at Austin
Austin, Texas

Contributors

Linda Stevens Albrecht, MBA, R.Ph., FASHP
Regional Director, Dallas/Fort Worth Region
College of Pharmacy
The University of Texas at Austin
Arlington, Texas

David D. Allen, R.Ph., Ph.D., FASHP
Dean and Professor
College of Pharmacy
Northeastern Ohio Universities
Rootstown, Ohio

Kristen Mizgate Bader, R.Ph.
Advanced Community Pharmacy Practice Coordinator
Austin/Temple/Waco Region
Clinical Instructor
Division of Pharmacy Practice
College of Pharmacy
University of Texas at Austin
Austin, Texas

Randy Ball, MBA, R.Ph.
Director of Pharmacy
Texas Health Harris Methodist Hospital Fort
  Worth
Fort Worth, Texas

Louis D. Barone, Pharm.D., R.Ph.
Vice Chair of Pharmacy Practice
Adjunct Assistant Professor
College of Pharmacy
Northeastern Ohio Universities
Rootstown, Ohio

Cindi Brennan, Pharm.D., MHA, FASHP
Director of Clinical Excellence
UW Medicine Pharmacy Services
Clinical Professor
University of Washington School of Pharmacy
Seattle, Washington

**Todd W. Canada, Pharm.D., BCNSP,
  FASHP**
Clinical Pharmacy Services Manager and Director
PGY-2 Critical Care/Nutrition Support
  Residency
Division of Pharmacy
University of Texas MD Anderson Cancer
  Center
Regional Internship Director
Galveston/Houston Region
College of Pharmacy
University of Texas at Austin
Houston, Texas

**Jannet M. Carmichael, Pharm.D., FCCP,
  FAPhA, BCPS**
VISN 21 Pharmacy Executive
PGY2 Residency Director
VA Sierra Pacific Network
Reno, Nevada

Cynthia A. Clegg, BS Pharm, MHA
Assistant Director
Ambulatory Pharmacy Services
Harborview Medical Center
Clinical Associate Professor
University of Washington School of Pharmacy
Seattle, Washington

Tammy Cohen, Pharm.D., MS
Director of Clinical Pharmacy Services
Baylor Health Care System
Director of Pharmacy
Baylor Heart & Vascular Hospital
Dallas, Texas

James Colbert, Jr., Pharm.D., FASHP
Associate Clinical Professor of Pharmacy
Assistant Dean for Experiential Education
Skaggs School of Pharmacy and Pharmaceutical Sciences
University of California, San Diego
La Jolla, California

Nicanora C. Cuéllar, MSW, LCSW, DCSW
Senior Social Worker
Pediatric Rheumatology Center
Texas Children's Hospital
Houston, Texas

Debra S. Devereaux, MBA, FASHP
Senior Consultant, Pharmacy Benefits
Gorman Health Group LLC
Washington, DC

Jordan F. Dow, Pharm.D., MS Candidate
Administrative Pharmacy Resident and Clinical Instructor
University of Wisconsin Hospital and Clinics
Madison, Wisconsin

Steven H. Dzierba, R.Ph., MS, FASHP
Medical Outcomes Specialist
Pfizer Global Medical
Southlake, Texas

Dale E. English II, R.Ph., Pharm.D., FASHP
Director, Instructional Labs
Adjunct Assistant Professor
Department of Pharmaceutical Sciences
Adjunct Assistant Professor
Department of Pharmacy Practice
Colleges of Medicine and Pharmacy
Northeastern Ohio Universities
Rootstown, Ohio

Dana S. Fitzsimmons, R.Ph., MBA, FASHP, MPH
Team Leader
Medical Outcomes Specialists
U.S. Medical Affairs
Pfizer, Inc.
Washington, DC

Bradi L. Frei, Pharm.D., BCOP, BCPS
Assistant Professor
Feik School of Pharmacy
University of the Incarnate Word
San Antonio, Texas

Molly E. Graham, Pharm.D.
Assistant Professor of Pharmacy Practice
Texas Tech University Health Sciences Center
School of Pharmacy
Abilene, Texas

Roy T. Hendley, MS, Pharm.D.
PGY1 Pharmacy Resident
Department of Pharmacy Services
The Methodist Hospital
Houston, Texas

William N. Jones, MS, R.Ph., FASHP
Pharmacy Program Manager for Educational Development
and Performance Improvement
Department of Veterans Affairs
Tucson, Arizona
Associate Clinical Professor
Department of Pharmacy Practice and Science
The College of Pharmacy
The University of Arizona
Tucson, Arizona

Grace M. Kuo, Pharm.D., MPH
UCSD Associate Professor of Clinical Pharmacy
UCSD Associate Adjunct Professor of Family and
Preventive Medicine
University of California, San Diego
La Jolla, California

Andrew Laegeler, MS, Pharm.D.
PGY1 Pharmacy Resident
St. Luke's Episcopal Hospital
Houston, Texas

Sarah E. Lake-Wallace, Pharm.D., MS
Director of Patient Safety and Performance Improvement
TIRR Memorial Hermann
Houston, Texas

David Lorms, CAE
President
Core Concept Solutions, LLC
Gaithersburg, Maryland

Darlene M. Mednick, R.Ph., MBA, Ph.D., FAMCP
Senior Vice President
Strategic Business Development, Managed Care
CareMed Pharmaceutical Services
Lake Success, New York

Traci L. Metting, Pharm.D., R.Ph.
Senior Director
The Preference Group™ (a division of Broadlane)
Dallas, Texas

John E. Murphy, Pharm.D., FCCP, FASHP
Professor of Pharmacy Practice and Science
Associate Dean
The University of Arizona College of Pharmacy
Tucson, Arizona

Ruth E. Nemire, BS Pharm., Pharm.D., Ed.D.
Associate Dean and Professor
Touro College of Pharmacy
New York, New York

Dehuti A. Pandya, Pharm.D, BCPS
Clinical Pharmacist—Brain Injury and Stroke
Program
TIRR Memorial Hermann Rehabilitation
and Research
Houston, Texas

Roland A. Patry, Dr.P.H., FASHP
Professor & Chair
Department of Pharmacy Practice
School of Pharmacy
Texas Tech University Health Sciences Center
Amarillo, Texas

Michael Piñón, Pharm.D.
Regional Scientific Associate Director
U.S. Medical & Drug Regulatory Affairs
Scientific Operations, Cardiovascular &
Metabolism
Novartis Pharmaceuticals Corporation
Houston, Texas

Vikki Jill Polk, Pharm.D.
Southwest Cancer Treatment and Research
Center
University Medical Center
Lubbock, Texas

Kevin Purcell, MD, Pharm.D., MHA, FIDSA, FASHP, FACHE
CHRISTUS Santa Rosa Health Care
Feik School of Pharmacy
University of the Incarnate Word
San Antonio, Texas

Jennifer L. Ridings-Myhra
Clinical Associate Professor
Assistant Dean for Experiential and Professional
Affairs
College of Pharmacy
The University of Texas at Austin
Austin, Texas

Michael D. Sanborn, MS, FASHP
Corporate Vice President for Cardiovascular
Services
Baylor Health Care System
Dallas, Texas

Margie E. Snyder, Pharm.D., MPH
Community Practice Research Fellow
University of Pittsburgh School of
    Pharmacy
Pittsburgh, Pennsylvania

Edward Stemley, MS, Pharm.D.
*Consultant in Health-System Pharmacy
    Administration*
Gulf Coast Region
Houston, Texas

**Stacy A. Taylor, Pharm.D., MHA,
    BCPS**
Pharmacy Clinical Manager
Cardinal Health/St. Joseph Health System
Bryan, Texas

Lee C. Vermeulen, R.Ph., MS, FCCP
Director, Center for Drug Policy
University of Wisconsin Hospital and
    Clinics
Clinical Associate Professor
UW—Madison School of Pharmacy
Madison, Wisconsin

Sara J. White, MS, FASHP
Pharmacy Leadership Coach
(Ret.) Director of Pharmacy
Stanford Hospital and Clinics
Stanford, California

Cynthia Wilson, BS Pharm., Pharm.D.
Manager, Pharmaceutical Services
St. Anthony Hospital
Franciscan Health System
Gig Harbor, Washington

Reviewers

**Angela Brownfield, Pharm.D., R.Ph.,
    BA**
Community Pharmacist
D & H Pharmacy
Columbia, Missouri
Adjunct Instructor of Pharmacy Practice
Community Pharmaceutical Care
St. Louis College of Pharmacy
Creighton University School of Pharmacy
University of Missouri-Kansas City School
    of Pharmacy
Kansas City, Missouri

**Raymond W. Hammond, Pharm.D.,
    BCPS**
Associate Dean for Practice Programs
University of Houston College of
    Pharmacy
Houston, Texas

Philip M. Hritcko, Pharm.D., CACP
Assistant Department Head
*Director, Experiential Education & Assistant
    Clinical Professor*
University of Connecticut School of
    Pharmacy
Storrs, Connecticut

Nancy A. Huff, Pharm.D.
Director of Pharmacy
Rehabilitation and Respiratory Services
Caritas Norwood Hospital
Norwood, Massachusetts

Erin Johanson, BS, M.Ed.
Assistant Director of Experiential Education
Midwestern University, College of
    Pharmacy-Glendale
Glendale, Arizona

**Anne Policastri, Pharm.D., MBA,
    FKSHP**
Assistant Director of Experiential Education
University of Kentucky College of
    Pharmacy
Lexington, Kentucky

If a teacher is indeed wise he does not bid you enter the house of his wisdom, but rather leads you to the threshold of your own mind.

Kahil Gibran

Preface

As children, we were both taught that people appreciate you far more for what you do and how you treat others, rather than for what you say you will do or for any material wealth you may have. How do you measure the worth of the outstanding preceptors and mentors that have come into our lives? Each one of us demonstrates or exemplifies characteristics or skills that we learned along the path toward becoming the pharmacists we are today.

Diane and I have been very fortunate to have significant influences in our lives that have guided our personal and professional development. There are many individuals that have contributed toward my development as a pharmacist and as an effective pharmacy manager and leader. While I was still in pharmacy school, my long time friend and colleague, Grace Salazar, and I were the first two women to work in the pharmacy at the VA Hospital in Houston. Back then as today, the VA was responsible for dispensing thousands of prescriptions for inpatients and outpatient veterans in our community on a daily basis. The pharmacists at the Houston VA taught me how to respond in a highly stressful environment, how to focus on one patient at a time regardless of the workload, how to communicate with empathy and understanding, and how to be part of a team. They set the bar high, guided me through the learning process, and always provided positive feedback.

From my brother, Celso Cuéllar, who is a long time community pharmacist, I learned how to talk to patients at a level they can understand in a respectful and culturally appropriate manner, how pharmacists can truly become extended members of many of their patients' families, and how empathy, kindness and good listening skills are often the best tools toward affecting compliance and effective medication management.

From the physicians, nurses, pharmacists, technicians, administrative support staff, and other colleagues at TIRR Memorial Hermann where I work, I have learned and continue to learn the true meaning of compassion, collaboration, and teamwork. Being an active member and officer of both my local and state health-system pharmacy organizations also gave me the opportunity to grow personally and professionally.

My colleagues and fellow directors of pharmacy in the Texas Medical Center and the Memorial Hermann Health System have facilitated my development as an effective pharmacy leader. We have shared experiences, sought advice from one another, and continue to collaborate on issues pertinent to the profession. From my friend, colleague, and coeditor of this book, Diane Ginsburg, I learned the art of networking and the value of becoming involved with professional organizations at the national level. In addition, she has given me numerous opportunities to develop and advance professionally. Her commitment to students and young practitioners as a teacher, counselor, mentor, and friend is truly commendable.

The need for proficient, energetic preceptors has never been greater. This edition, like the first, is designed to provide pharmacists with critical information about preceptor programs around the U.S. and to help preceptors design a dynamic and effective experiential program at their practice site. We have identified topics that we felt would be important for preceptors at all levels and sites of practice (hospital, community, industry, faculty, etc.). We have added several topics to this edition including examples of assessment tools, competencies, and goals and objectives for different rotations. This book is meant to be comprehensive, and topics and sections are organized by common areas of skills or proficiencies.

To be an effective preceptor, a pharmacist should exhibit clinical competency skills, possess excellent written and verbal communication skills, and also demonstrate humanistic skills such as listening, compassion, empathy, and observation. Diane Ginsburg and I invited pharmacists from around the U.S. that exemplify the characteristics of exemplary preceptors. In addition, authors were invited who had expertise in their respective areas and brought perspective from different parts of the country and different or unique practice programs. The intent is for this book to be reflective on broad practice guidelines.

One of the greatest satisfactions you can have as a pharmacist today is mentoring students and young practitioners. I am still in contact with the very first student I had the privilege to precept. It is hard to express into words the pride and satisfaction one feels as students you have mentored and precepted develop into outstanding professionals and clinicians.

How do you measure the worth of exemplary preceptors and mentors? You cannot. You thank them for their selfless contributions by practicing and enhancing the skills and training they provided to you. Most importantly, you pass these gifts on to the next generation of practitioners.

Lourdes M. Cuéllar
March 2009

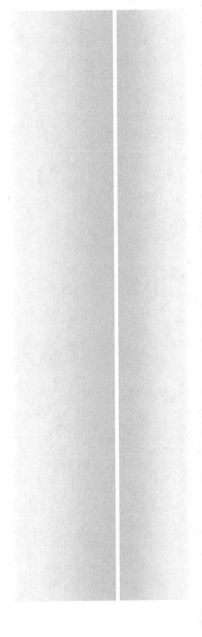

Modeling may not only be the best way to teach, it may be the only way to teach.
Albert Schweitzer

Chapter 1

Precepting Fundamentals

Sara J.White, Kevin Purcell, Randy Ball, Lourdes M. Cuéllar

Chapter Outline

Learning Objectives

- Define precepting and mentoring.
- Create activities that provide students with the opportunity to meet all learning objectives while meeting work requirements.
- Define and discuss the main areas of focus for preceptors.
- Identify technical skills and abilities for preceptors.
- Identify core values of preceptors.

Being an effective preceptor is a significant professional responsibility, different from being a competent pharmacist. You must have an understanding of precepting and have outlined your duties. Since precepting involves one-on-one communication, interpersonal and teaching skills are very important. Even a seasoned preceptor must continue to improve his or her skills. This chapter defines precepting and mentoring and discusses some of the basics of successful precepting.

Origins of Precepting and Mentoring

The theories of precepting and mentoring have existed for a long time and can be traced back to ancient Greece and Greek mythology. Precepting can be defined as teaching students the art and science of practice in a healthcare setting (e.g., in the context of pharmacy, precepting would occur in a community pharmacy, a hospital, a clinic, etc.) with the goal of developing competent practitioners. The earliest reference to precepting can be found in the Hippocratic oath written around 400 B.C. by the great Greek physician Hippocrates (Box 1.1).[1,2] In his famous oath, Hippocrates defined a set of very compelling duties and responsibilities of the physician, which can be applied to preceptors as well. A strong and enduring commitment to patient care was formed as the art of medicine was passed down from father to son and from preceptor to student. Today, the science of pharmacy is taught in universities, but the art is still passed on from preceptor to student.

The word mentor comes from *The Odyssey*, written in approximately 700 B.C. by the Greek poet Homer.[3] Mentor was the name of a wise and loyal advisor and friend of Odysseus, the King of Ithaca. During the 20 years Odysseus was gone fighting in the Trojan War and traveling home, he entrusted Mentor with his household and the direction and teaching of his son, Telemachus. Mentoring is now defined as helping others reach their full potential as professionals with the goal of developing practitioners who will pursue and attain excellence as patient care providers, teachers, scientists, managers, and/or leaders.

Box 1.1 • Hippocratic Oath[1,2]

I swear by Apollo Physician and Asclepios and Hygeia and Panacea and all the gods and goddesses, making them my witnesses, that I will fulfill according to my ability and judgment this oath and this covenant:

To hold him who has taught me this art as equal to my parents and to live my life in partnership with him, and if he is in need of money to give him a share of mine, and to regard his offspring as equal to my brothers in male lineage and to teach them this art—if they desire to learn it—without fee and covenant; to give a share of precepts and oral instruction and all other learning to my sons and to the sons of him who has instructed me and to the pupils who have signed the covenant and have taken an oath according to the medical law, but to no one else.

I will apply dietetic measures for the benefit of the sick according to my ability and judgment; I will keep them from harm and injustice.

I will neither give a deadly drug to anybody if asked for it, nor will I make a suggestion to this effect. Similarly, I will not give to a woman an abortive remedy. In purity and holiness I will guard my life and my art.

I will not use the knife, not even on sufferers from stone, but will withdraw in favor of such men as are engaged in this work.

Whatever houses I may visit, I will come for the benefit of the sick, remaining free of all intentional injustice, of all mischief, and in particular of sexual relations with both female and male persons, be they free or slaves.

What I may see or hear in the course of treatment or even outside of the treatment in regard to the life of men, which on no account one must spread abroad, I will keep to myself, holding such things shameful to be spoken about.

If I fulfill this oath and do not violate it, may it be granted to me to enjoy life and art, being honored with fame among all men for all time to come; if I transgress it and swear falsely, may the opposite of all this be my lot.

Today the concepts of precepting and mentoring are vital to the professional growth and development of pharmacy students and pharmacists and to the future of the pharmacy profession. We rely on experienced practitioners to become preceptors and to pass down knowledge and experience to their preceptees. Precepting involves a partnership for education, investment of time and energy, negotiation and individualization of learning activities, teamwork, coaching, evaluation of performance, and professionalism role modeling and guidance (Box 1.2). Preceptors ensure that their preceptees attain competency at the practice of pharmacy much in the same way that master craftsmen supervise apprentices in developing the skills of their trade. Service is exchanged for education and training.

Box 1.2 • The Elements of Precepting[1,2]

Partnership

Role modeling

Education

Coaching

Evaluation

Professionalism

Teamwork

Investment

Negotiation

Guidance

After a student finishes the formal precepting from their academic process, he or she may then choose a mentor to utilize as a pharmacist. Mentoring is a relationship based on the following: trust and respect; education and nurturing; inspiration to advance the practice of pharmacy and improve patient care; opportunities to grow and develop; metamorphosis through engaging in a process of self-reflection, self-assessment, and self-transformation; professional guidance; and nomination for awards when success has been achieved (Box 1.3). We depend on preceptors to also become mentors and to help their mentees attain professional excellence and become leaders. Pharmacy preceptors and mentors provide the most critical aspects of professional education and training and truly can make a difference in the lives and careers of their preceptees and mentees.

Box 1.3 • The Elements of Mentoring[1,2]

Metamorphosis

Education

Nurturing

Trust

Opportunity

Respect

Inspiration

Nomination

Guidance

Preceptor: A Job Description

While the State Boards of Pharmacy define the legal responsibilities of preceptors, and the colleges and schools of pharmacy define the educational requirements of the rotation, precepting requires many skills and traits that these formal bodies do not identify. Preceptors are responsible for the education of students while on rotation, but this education is not the didactic, lecturer-student relationship of the classroom environment. Two of the most important areas of focus for preceptors include teaching students how to be professionals and teaching them how to apply the knowledge they have gained from didactic courses in real, dynamic patient care situations. To achieve this goal, preceptors must possess a set of core values, technical skills, and abilities.

• Preceptor Pearls •

Preceptors teach students how to be professionals and how to apply their knowledge in clinical situations.

The core values for a preceptor include the following:

- Professionalism. Students learn to be professionals not from textbooks but rather by observing practitioners in the experiential setting and by functioning as healthcare providers themselves. The most important person to instill this professionalism in students is the preceptor. To do so, the preceptor must exhibit professional behavior and discuss professional issues with students. The preceptor should also discuss professional organizations with students and encourage students to become active members in these organizations.
- Desire to educate and share knowledge with students.
- Willingness to mentor. The progression of students from the classroom setting to experiential sites and, ultimately, to professional practice requires personal growth of the students. Preceptors must be willing to serve as mentors to their students, guiding them along their path from students to pharmacists and helping them move from an educational model of student/teacher to mentor/mentee. This transition will prepare students for the lifetime learning model that all pharmacists follow.
- Willingness to commit the time necessary for precepting. The majority of experiential rotations are supervised by pharmacists who are precepting students while performing their normal duties. Teaching while maintaining a full work schedule requires preceptors to have a true desire to teach and to commit the time necessary to teach. Precepting often requires a time commitment beyond normal working hours. Without the true desire to educate students and the willingness to devote the necessary time, preceptors will not be able to effectively teach their preceptees.
- Respect for others
- Willingness to work with a diverse student population. The student population today is more diverse than it was even 10 years ago. This diversity includes ethnic and gender diversity, along with cultural and generational diversity. Many students today are entering pharmacy school after having worked for several years in another profession, and many

students already possess advanced degrees in other fields. While these factors will help strengthen the pharmacy profession in the future, preceptors must recognize and respect these differences. The degree of diversity that exists today also requires preceptors to adapt teaching techniques for maximizing students' learning experiences. When precepting multiple students on the same rotation, diversity factors can present unique and challenging situations.

While each preceptor will have different areas of strength within these core values, the preceptor must hold each of these values as personally important.

Additionally, precepting students on experiential rotations requires excellent skills in the relevant subject area. If a preceptor is not knowledgeable about a particular area, students will not gain the necessary oversight and guidance to meet their learning objectives. A rotation with an unprepared or inexperienced preceptor can also adversely affect the students' view of the profession. Preceptors should never be forced to take students on a rotation if they are not competent in that particular area. Sometimes—in an effort to schedule an experiential rotation for students—the site will try to accommodate both the students' and the college's needs. When this occurs, the site and preceptor almost always fall short, and the result is a negative experience for all involved.

As stated above, precepting is an additional duty that a pharmacist takes on because of the desire to be involved in the educational process of our profession. To be effective at balancing the requirements of the job with time spent teaching, preceptors must possess a number of abilities. They must have good written and oral communication skills, and good organizational and time management skills. Knowledge of resource utilization requirements of the site is also helpful in achieving the balance between the practice and precepting, potentially allowing preceptors to work within these resource requirements to involve others in the process.

• Preceptor Pearls •

A preceptor must have good communication, organizational, and time management skills.

Why Being a Preceptor Is an Important Aspect of Pharmacy Practice

The practice of pharmacy is a proud profession with a rich history and many varied practice settings. The future of pharmacy will be determined by recent and future graduates. These graduates rely heavily on experiential rotations for developing their foundation in pharmacy practice today and what it can be in the future.

Each practice setting has unique experiences that can be utilized to teach students how to practice pharmacy in a real world environment. Through experiential rotations, students learn how to apply the knowledge they have acquired in their pharmacy school coursework. Students also learn how to be professionals and how to interact with other healthcare practitioners. Precepted experiential rotations provide students with the opportunity to learn how to provide pharmaceutical care within various practice settings, while under the guidance of a skilled practitioner.

In addition to the value precepting has for the students, precepting rotations also provides value to the practice site. Hosting students on experiential rotations provides the site with an infusion of intelligent practitioners who help to keep the pharmacy knowledge base sharpened. Journal clubs and formal presentations provide pharmacy staff, both professional and technical, with up-to-date pharmacy information. Students who have completed interesting rotations also serve as positive advertising for the pharmacy among their classmates as they begin to seek employment after graduation.

In addition to the benefit to students and training sites, precepting is also professionally rewarding for preceptors. They have the opportunity to influence future practitioners and, in doing so, can influence the future of the profession for many years to come. Precepting also helps sharpen preceptors, as they reinforce their own knowledge and expand their own horizons through student interactions. As preceptors answer questions and explain pharmacy practice, they gain an even deeper understanding of their own practice. Routine daily tasks that preceptors frequently do without much thought become fresh again as they explain them to students. Taking time to befriend students also creates a unique professional bond that can last beyond the rotation period. It is not uncommon for former students to maintain contact with preceptors who helped to shape their professional perspective.

• Preceptor Pearls •

Precepting benefits both the student and the preceptor, who learn from each other.

Overall and when done correctly, precepting experiential rotations is one of the most important aspects of pharmacy practice. When the time and resources are devoted to making the rotation a top notch experience, the students, the preceptor, and the site all benefit. Ultimately, patient care is improved, and this is the reason we practice pharmacy.

New Ideas for Seasoned Preceptors

Seasoned preceptors often like to experiment with implementing new ideas and concepts into their internship programs. This provides some new challenges and excitement for preceptors as well as some new learning opportunities for students. Preceptors can either formulate unique and innovative ideas that are true revolutionary advances in student education, or they can simply add a different spin to the ideas and practices of others. This section of the chapter presents ideas that both new and seasoned preceptors can use to help students to become the best pharmacists they can be.

• Preceptor Pearls •

Incorporating unique activities into a rotation ensures both the student and the preceptor remain engaged and committed.

Competency Portfolio

One idea is for preceptors to require students to assemble a competency portfolio during the internship that documents their competency in the desired areas. This would be consistent with the movement in healthcare to better assess the competency of students, residents, and practitioners with the ultimate goal of improving patient safety and outcomes (clinical, economic, and humanistic). Competency is difficult to assess because it is composed of multiple domains, including knowledge, skills, abilities, values, attitudes, beliefs, and behaviors. No single evaluation method (e.g., examinations, assignments, direct observation, etc.) can be used to accurately and appropriately assess competency in all of these areas. Competency assessment really requires the use of a variety of methods and instruments.

A comprehensive competency portfolio may have some similarity to a diary (e.g., reflective writing on feelings and experiences) and also to a promotion and/or tenure dossier of a faculty member (e.g., demonstration of activity and achievement in certain areas, including practice, teaching, research, and service). Of course, the first step is to define the desired areas of competency for students. Preceptors should check with their respective academic programs to determine if the programs require identification of the desired areas of competency, and then incorporate it into their experiential program. The pharmacy schools with which preceptors are affiliated may have already done this. If not, preceptors can take the lead and develop a set of competencies that they expect students to have after completion of their internship. The Accreditation Council for Graduate Medical Education required by June 2006 that all medical and surgical residency programs implement methods to assess and document competency of their graduates in the following six areas: patient care, medical knowledge, practice-based learning and improvement, interpersonal and communication skills, professionalism, and systems-based practice.[4] Also, the American Association of Colleges of Pharmacy has developed its own set of educational outcomes.[5] As the preceptor, you could develop a list of some example pharmacy practice competencies that you could further define and use to assess students. Students can demonstrate how each competency has been attained through a variety of documents in a competency portfolio as well as by doing some self-assessment and reflective writing related to each competency. Each competency could have its own section in a three-ring binder, and the same binder could probably contain the internship manual (the internship syllabus and other useful information) and the competency portfolio materials.

Using Artistic Media as a Teaching Tool

Preceptors might find ways to apply art, music, poetry, and literature to pharmacy practice and student education in order to help students develop their humanistic qualities and broaden their cultural education. Some art, music, poetry, and literature can portray an expression of the artist's/ author's feelings and experiences with disease, the healthcare system, and society. Using artistic media for teaching purposes can help students see illness and treatment from their patients' perspectives and comprehend their patients' suffering so that they can accompany them through illnesses with empathy, respect, and effective care. Studying and trying to interpret art, music, poetry, and literature also can help sharpen observational skills (seeing what is present and not present) and listening skills (hearing what patients are really saying). Although it can be difficult to detect subtle meaning in pictures and phrases, it can be just as difficult to understand the significance of the tone of a patient's words, the inflection of his/her voice, and his/her facial expressions and body language.

There are multiple ways to incorporate the visual or performing arts as well as literature and poetry into an internship, and preceptors are only limited by their own creativity and artistic ability. Critically evaluating artwork, especially paintings and photographs of people, can enhance and hone observational skills.[6] A trip to a local art museum could be incorporated into the internship and could occur on the weekend.

Alternatively, art books or slides could be used at the practice site, but doing so may lose some of the culturally enhancing atmosphere. The most powerful aspect of physical examination is observation. One can obtain a lot of relevant medical information just from carefully observing someone, describing what is seen, and interpreting the findings. Observing, describing, and interpreting artwork can help develop these skills. Revealing the history of the artwork and what the artists meant to convey can complete the exercise.

Also, patients have written many books and poems about coping with their diseases. Students could be required to read some selected books and poems to better understand patients' perspectives. Seeing things through patients' eyes may make students appreciate the strength of a holistic model of patient care that addresses the mind, body, and spirit and considers all the various factors that affect health and well-being[7,8] Often healthcare professionals focus only on treating patients' diseases (the physical aspect) but ignore psychological, spiritual, socioeconomic, cultural, and environmental factors that affect their patients' healthcare outcomes. Finally, reading essays, poems, and books written by pharmacists or other practitioners may also help students understand what it means to be a pharmacist and a healthcare professional.

Creating a Practice Model

Preceptors can create a practice model for students with defined duties and responsibilities that are important functions and aspects of patient care and pharmacy operations. Often students do not have clearly defined roles at practice sites, and they are not well integrated into the patient care process or the pharmacy operations. Of course, it is hard for preceptors to essentially create an unsalaried job position and a job description for students if they do not have a constant supply of students. Student intern positions with important duties and responsibilities would have to be filled year-round to provide consistency and continuity of services, especially if the students are integrated into a patient care unit and team in a hospital. Once expectations of other healthcare professionals have been built and met by students providing them support for patient care services, there cannot be lapses in coverage. The practice site will need to always have a student in that position. This will require a strong partnership with one or more pharmacy schools in order to meet the site's demand for students.

For example, under the supervision of a pharmacist preceptor, students can be decentralized to a patient care unit or to a team in a hospital and provide a spectrum of pharmacy services. Students could be responsible for a number of functions including taking initial medication histories; conducting daily drug regimen reviews; answering drug information questions; performing therapeutic drug monitoring services; writing patient care plans and daily progress notes; reviewing discharge medications; counseling patients; and providing inservices to the medical, nursing, and allied health staff. Students also could act as liaisons for the pharmacy department and help nurses on the patient care units and centralized staff pharmacists troubleshoot problems with the medication use system (prescribing, dispensing, administration, and monitoring). Students can be provided a pager so that the unit, team, and preceptor can always reach them.

Although the above example is for creating a student practice model in an inpatient unit, student practice models related to patient care services or pharmacy operations and management could be developed in many other pharmacy practice settings. Also, when at all possible, preceptors should get senior students involved in more advanced practice activities and involve other professionals (e.g., physicians, nurses, dietitians, respiratory therapists, business managers) in their internships as co-preceptors to provide more diverse education and experiences. Advanced practice activities can include disease screenings; patient assessment (physical examination, laboratory test interpretation, etc.); medication administration; drug therapy and disease management; patient counseling on health promotion/disease prevention and on their specific diseases and medications; and practice and financial management. Additionally, students could act as teachers by providing inservices to healthcare professions and educating support groups about drug therapy and disease management. Teaching is a very effective way to ensure a full understanding of the material.

Publication

Preceptors can encourage students to present and publish their work on projects or their opinions on issues. Presenting and publishing are excellent educational activities, and they also bring recognition. There are numerous opportunities for students to present (e.g., local, state, and national pharmacy society meetings, community organization meetings) or publish (e.g., employer or professional society newsletters, local and national newspapers, state and national pharmacy society journals) their work or opinions. Often students are required to complete a project (e.g., research, process improvement, community service, etc.) or an assignment (e.g., formulary monograph, therapeutic review, etc.) that they could present or publish in a variety of forums. Also, students sometimes see patients with significant clinical findings that are either unusual or new and not previously reported, which they could write up as a brief case report. They can submit their thoughts on issues as viewpoints, opinions, commentaries, or letters to the editor to many newsletters, newspapers, and journals. They can also write a review article for a newsletter or journal based on background research they have done for finding answers to patient care problems, the development of policies and procedures, or the conducting of formulary evaluations. Overall, writing articles of any type can reinforce learning, enhance written communication skills, and stimulate one to clarify his/her beliefs and positions.

Professional Societies and Community Service Organizations

Preceptors are often involved in professional societies and community service organizations but sometimes fail to get students involved, especially since the meetings tend to be in the evenings and the activities are usually on the weekends. However, preceptors need to take students with them to these functions. Participation in professional societies and community service organizations is a critical element of the professionalization process and provides one of the best opportunities for leadership development.

Preceptors do not need to give students compensatory time off during the workweek for attending evening and weekend professional society and community service activities. Preceptors do not get compensatory time off from work for doing this, so students do not either. This is part of the students' learning about the life of a pharmacist who is dedicated to public service, to the advancement of pharmacy practice and patient care, and to lifelong learning. Some colleges of pharmacy recognize attendance of outside professional organizational meetings as "Special Activity Hours" and give credit for these during the rotation.

Summary

Preceptors must keep in mind that more than anything else students want to be able to spend quality time talking with and learning from them. Often because of the hectic nature of many practice environments, preceptors are not able to spare much time during the workday to do this. One way to accommodate this desire and need of students for their preceptors' time is to set aside time outside of the workday. For example, preceptors could have a cup of coffee or breakfast with students every Friday morning before work. The topics for discussion could be left up to the students since this is their time with their preceptors. Topics could encompass everything from deciding on an initial career pathway and getting a job to discussing how to proactively address issues facing the profession though advocacy and leadership.

These are just a few of an infinite number of ideas and concepts that can be used to add value to an internship program and make the educational process more meaningful and fulfilling to both preceptors and students. It is important for preceptors to keep themselves challenged, excited, and energized about precepting students. Experimenting with ways to add new dimensions to internships or to completely reinvent internships can be therapeutic for preceptors and can create new and better learning opportunities for students.

Integrating Pharmacy Students into Your Practice

Pharmacy education in most practice settings is characterized in part by balancing educational effectiveness, while simultaneously trying to provide optimal patient care. As practitioners we are all juggling multiple tasks and responsibilities while teaching and supervising students. Time constraints and multiple pressures and deadlines are all factors that today's practitioners face. The constraints associated with high census, high volume, high patient acuity, clarifying prescriptions or medication orders, dealing with insurance problems, and staffing shortages only serve to escalate the intensity of dealing with all the important aspects of being an effective preceptor. There are educationally sound methods that incorporate time management, organizational skills, service learning, and effective planning to assist preceptors in integrating pharmacy student education and meeting employment and practice requirements.

Be prepared when students arrive at your facility or practice setting. Students appreciate structure, and it provides them with the opportunity not only to meet all learning objectives but also to be trained and participate in services and activities that are unique to your practice setting. As the preceptor you will be able to teach in a more productive manner and allow the students to have effective patient encounters with appropriate education, guidance, and supervision.

Begin by developing a training manual specific to your facility and experiential rotation(s). This demonstrates to the students your commitment to their education and training. Be creative when developing your manual. Be innovative with the content of the manual. For example use business articles to teach negotiation skills. Insert materials that the student can keep and those that are a permanent part of the manual. Use puzzles and medical artwork to help train, test, and reinforce skills and competency.

Begin with a welcome letter or memo. In the manual, be sure to include not only information about the pharmacy and the experiential rotation, but also information about your hospital, community pharmacy, ambulatory care site, specialty site, or other practice site or facility. Do not forget to include a map of your facility, especially if it is a large teaching or community hospital. Tell the story of your institution. Include organizational maps of the hospital or practice site and of your department. Insert a copy of your job description as well as other position descriptions that may be of interest to the student. Students who have never worked in a pharmacy or seen a pharmacist in clinical practice are often surprised at the extent of duties and responsibilities and the creative practice structure of pharmacists in today's health system, community practice, ambulatory care, management, and other professional practice environments.

• Preceptor Pearls •

Providing students with a detailed training manual on their first day begins to orient students to the training site and shows you are committed to their training.

Orienting the students to the training site is a well-recognized strategy for creating a positive learning experience and communicating goals, objectives, and minimal competencies for the experiential training rotation. Orientation should include the following:

- Goals, objectives, and minimal competency requirements of the rotation
- Rotation hours and attendance policy
- Any requirements of the student during off-hours
- Regulatory compliance standards relating to your State Board of Pharmacy
- Tour of your facility and department
- Review of required reading for the rotation
- Terms and definitions for students completing a rotation in an unfamiliar practice setting
- A trip to Human Resources to obtain an identification badge and complete facility orientation requirements (e.g., infection control, HIPAA)
- Introduction to all members of the department or practice and a brief explanation of their duties
- Introduction to key members of the medical, nursing, and other health professional staff, or store or office manager with whom the student will be working on a day-to-day basis; in a community setting, it is also helpful to include a listing of the top physician prescribers.

- A review of the facility's policies and procedures
- Introduction to your pharmacy information system and insurance adjudication system
- An introduction to your site's drug utilization review process
- Introduction or review of your facility-specific medical record system or patient information system
- A list of your community practice's "fast movers"
- Review of all pertinent medication use policies (e.g., standard administration times, approved abbreviations, and substitution guidelines), including how errors are handled
- Publications, journals, and other reference materials available to students
- Evaluation instruments, timing and methods, exams and grading policy

You will need to devote a significant amount of time the first week of the rotation to setting expectations and ground rules. By ensuring that students have a full understanding of your expectations, there is less of a chance for misinterpretation or confusion later. This also makes for an easier transition to empower students to take on projects and be more independent as they move throughout the remaining weeks of the rotation, with ongoing supervision and follow-up from the preceptor.

When building the schedule for the rotation, include time for preceptor teaching and feedback, and also time for the students to reflect on their patient encounters. Be sure to include midterm and final exam dates, site-specific and school events and holidays, and assignment due dates (e.g., case presentations, journal club, patient care plan: build in a project where the patients are sure to benefit and students experience success). Be sure to communicate your specific expectations to students.

Capitalize on the advantages of your practice site and your strengths as a preceptor when developing student schedules. Assign special projects and presentations that will benefit both the site and students. Include patient education, literature searches, physician case conferences, morbidity and mortality rounds, pharmacy and therapeutics or formulary meetings, grand rounds, and health screenings and immunization opportunities in community and ambulatory setting as part of their experiential training. As you review the schedule with students, be sure to allow them time to ask questions and take time to explain to them how all the activities impact patient care.

Allow for student individuality and creativity. Make provisions in the schedule to allow for activities that meet specific student needs and desires. Assess their strengths and weaknesses and allow enough flexibility to meet their educational needs and interests. If you develop a project encompassing some of their interests, they will be more motivated to perform those activities that are less interesting as well. Be flexible and try out new concepts or ideas. Most importantly, identify opportunities for student involvement when considering any and all of your planned activities.

Familiarize yourself with students' prior rotations, experiences, and professional goals. Assess the students' areas of interest. Determine their short- and long-term goals on day one of the rotation. Let them know that the schedule is flexible enough to allow for their involvement and input into planning their daily activities. Assess their readiness and motivation to learn. Ascertain if they have previous experience working as a pharmacy technician either in the hospital or retail setting. For example, students may have prior experience working as an IV technician in a health-system setting.

You may choose to perform a validation of their skills and then take the time normally assigned to that activity and change it to an area of particular interest to the students or on a special project or assignment. A student who has worked as a technician in a retail setting may have a comfort level with insurance adjudication and could work on health screenings and intake information projects instead.

• Preceptor Pearls •

Use students' experience, goals, and interests to help tailor the rotation to each student.

Students generally progress through predictable stages of learning development. It is critical to the success of the rotation that preceptors take time on the first days of the rotation to assess each student individually. This exercise should not only determine students' basic pharmacological competency and core clinical and patient encounter skills, but also verbal and written communication skills, problem solving skills, and ability to perform multiple tasks and handle complex patients. As a preceptor you should be able to rapidly identify student strengths and needs relative to meeting all the learning objectives of your rotation. Have a plan, but be flexible in adjusting to meet student needs and abilities.

The first meeting with your students sets the tone for the entire training encounter. Ensure that students understand and accept that both of you must work together throughout the rotation to assure quality patient care as well as quality education and training.

To have a successful experiential rotation, it is essential that the preceptor establishes standards. Be specific when you communicate your expectations to students. Offer students ideas as you mutually establish specific goals for their rotation. Give them creative challenges; promote their strengths. By linking the students' performance to those standards, the preceptor creates a benchmark for achievement. The ultimate goal is to transition from a teacher/student learner relationship to clinical supervisor/responsible performer (clinician) relationship. Students should be able to demonstrate their problem-solving skills and integrate their didactic knowledge and clinical training to real daily situations. There should be a good balance between education and service learning.

• Preceptor Pearls •

Establish standards and communicate them clearly to your students.

A good preceptor should be able to relate to students how all their activities impact patient care. Preceptors should provide guidance, answer questions, explain answers, and assist students in developing self-confidence and self-esteem. An exemplary preceptor demonstrates a positive attitude and is dedicated to helping students achieve their full potential.

Most experiential training sites afford students the opportunity to work and train with a number of other professionals besides the primary preceptor. Choose professionals who are motivated and committed to student education. The pharmacist team of preceptors can teach students a number of critical skills that are not necessarily related to the science of pharmacy but rather the human side of our profession. Students will also be able to observe different approaches taken by the various healthcare professionals. Some of these critical skills include ethics, teamwork, leadership skills, empathy and compassion, and communication, as well as the technical and cognitive abilities of being a pharmacist. Introduce diverse activities that provide students with the opportunity to meet all learning objectives while meeting work requirements.

In order to be able to simultaneously provide a successful educational experience and ensure clinical effectiveness, the preceptor must be organized and must identify strategies for providing educational opportunities. Orienting students to patient encounters is an effective strategy for creating a good learning environment and providing effective direct patient care. Learn to present a 1- to 2-minute patient-specific orientation. This will help students obtain a conceptual framework that will help them to efficiently interpret vital patient information. For example, the preceptor should review the patient's medical background; explain to students on which symptoms or conditions they should focus and how to look for nonverbal forms of communication by the patient; and establish guidelines for interventions, monitoring, or a patient care plan. Another example would be going over with students the importance of calling a physician if they are unclear about a prescription, the steps to take if they come across a drug interaction, or how to negotiate or talk with an angry patient or physician. During each patient-specific encounter, the preceptor should alert students to any potentially coexisting problems or additional medical conditions in the patient's history.

The patient case presentation or the drug utilization review process offer both the preceptor and students an optimal opportunity for teaching and learning. In addition, teaching with the patient allows the preceptor to observe students' performance and provide immediate feedback. The preceptor should verbally identify what students did well, and then ascertain problem areas and suggest steps students might take to correct them, without dictating a solution, even if it seems obvious. Box 1.4 lists some examples of effective opportunities to teach in a productive manner.

Remember that students should be active participants. The preceptor must take care not to make any pertinent learning activities a mere "shadowing" experience unless you are precepting an introductory pharmacy practice experience. Students should know the reason or rationale for all activities or projects.

Promote self-directed and life-long learning. At the end of the day ask the student, "What did you learn today?" or "What medical problem or condition would you like to learn more about?" or "What was the most important thing you learned today?" Link self-directed learning to a recently observed patient problem or departmental process or procedure. Self-directed learning can also include research, literature review, or selected reading about a disease or condition that is prevalent in the patient population you serve. Self-directed learning should apply the students' didactic knowledge to real-life patient encounters or experiences.

Service-based education is a very effective teaching tactic. There are two ways a preceptor can use this teaching strategy. The first is by identifying to students the tasks that are routinely performed by nonlicensed staff in your department or other healthcare providers. The second is by encouraging students to participate in community service-based education.

Nonlicensed staff is an integral part of the day-to-day operation of a pharmacy. To help students comprehend and appreciate how each employee is a valuable member of the pharmacy team, allow students to spend some time with the support staff within the department. During institutional and

Box 1.4 • Examples of Effective Opportunities to Teach in a Productive Manner

- Patient education and counseling
- Health screenings
- Pharmacotherapy, nutrition, renal dosing, and pharmacokinetic consults
- Literature searches
- Physician case conference or grand rounds presentations
- Patient-specific drug utilization review
- Performance enhancement activities such as evaluation of regulatory compliance
- MUE/DUE criteria development, data collection, queries, and compilation of results
- Interdisciplinary training (e.g., shadowing a nurse, dietician, or respiratory therapist for a set number of hours)
- Technician activities
- Departmental budget preparation and review process
- Employee feedback and evaluation process
- Policies and procedures development or revisions and updates to staff
- Patient case presentation
- Presentation for Pharmacy & Therapeutics Committee
- Journal club
- Drug information questions
- In-services for nurses, pharmacists, medical residents, and other disciplines and community
- Special projects, presentations, or experiences

community rotations, have them perform duties such as triaging patient or nursing phone calls, assisting at the service window, calling insurance companies, retrieving charts, repackaging medications, calling physicians to clarify orders, and assisting in the ordering and inventory process. It is also important for students to learn how these functions are critical to the operations of the department.

It is also imperative that students learn the value of community service education as part of their experiential training. Start by inviting them to go with you to one of your local pharmacy organizations' continuing education programs. Teach them the value of fellowship and networking with colleagues within your community.

• Preceptor Pearls •

Teach students the importance of community service.

If you are actively involved in any volunteer community activities, such as local health fairs, providing healthcare to the homeless, serving food at local shelters, or volunteering at a clinic for indigent families, invite the students to go with you. Alternatively, develop a community service site directory and let students choose where they would like to visit. Box 1.5 lists examples of good learning environments for students. Give them specific goals, such as learning about topics listed in Box 1.6. Also give them observation questions or assignments. Help them to see the "big picture" of healthcare as well as the specifics of patient care. Box 1.7 lists some examples of these questions and assignments.

The most useful activity after community service education is reflection. Focus on a teaching point, such as whether the student effectively addressed the patient's concerns. The preceptor should provide meaningful feedback and ask if the expectations were realistic and reasonable for the students. The goal is to help students realize that the contributions they can make go beyond the workplace environment. The professional rewards of the service-oriented teaching are great, and students recognize the value of intrinsic rewards such as personal and professional growth and development.

Find opportunities to ask students questions about their learning experience, such as in the cafeteria at lunch time. Provide frequent assessment; informal assessment should be ongoing throughout the rotation. In your informal conversations discuss issues such as lifetime learning habits, the role of residency training, balancing career and family goals, applying for a job, and interview skills.

Sit down with students at least once a week to provide formal feedback and assessment. Review the progress that they have made and give them the opportunity to come up with ways to improve areas that they need to strengthen. Be candid. Provide honest and constructive feedback. Listen carefully to students when you ask them for their self-assessment.

• Preceptor Pearls •

Provide frequent, specific, and constructive feedback.

Acknowledge student contributions. Do so in front of other members of the healthcare team or during a departmental staff meeting. This will go a long way in helping build self-esteem. Help them promote their strengths and teach them to assume broader responsibilities in meeting their educational goals.

Do not forget to bring in some real life experiences. Tell them about your preceptors and mentors and the influence they had on your life. As much as possible, be accessible and approachable to the students.

Summary

Both the preceptor and the students must be committed to patient care and to pharmacy education. The preceptor must consistently demonstrate competency and professionalism and have a passion for education, service, and excellence. Consistency and standardization are essential for effective

Box 1.5 • Examples of Service Learning Environments

- Adult or Child Protective Services
- Nursing home care unit
- City/county clinics or emergency room
- Visiting nurse association
- Hospital social work department
- Hospital chaplaincy
- Child development in a pediatric unit
- Local AIDS clinic
- Local substance abuse program

Box 1.6 • Examples of Topics Taught Through Service Learning

- The role of community agencies, nursing homes, hospices, and public agencies, programs, and clinics
- Professionalism and community spirit and advocacy
- How community health services are funded
- How to practice preventative medicine
- The social, economic, and ethical aspects of healthcare
- How a person's culture, heath beliefs and literacy level create health disparities and impact health outcomes

Box 1.7 • Examples of Questions and Assignments for Encouraging Observation in Service Learning Experiences

- What services are provided to the patient?
- List the disciplines and their roles within the clinic or facility.
- How do pharmacists interact with this site?
- Name some ways in which literacy is a public health issue.
- Identify common reasons why a physician orders home health or hospice care.
- List physical findings consistent with domestic violence or abuse.
- Describe the role of the hospital chaplain.
- Briefly define the care rendered at a skilled nursing facility and the role of the pharmacist.

teaching and integrating pharmacy students into your practice. Effective planning, comprehensive student orientation, setting clear expectations, introducing diverse learning experiences, and ongoing constructive feedback are integral to the students' successful learning experience.

References

1.   Edelstein L. The genuine works of Hippocrates. *Bull Hist Med*. 1939;7:236–8.

2.   Edelstein L. The Hippocratic oath: text, translation, and interpretation. *Bull Hist Med*. 1943;(suppl 1).

3.   Homer. *The Odyssey*. Translated by Rieu EV. London, England: Penguin Books; 1946.

4.   Accreditation Council for Graduate Medical Education. Outcome Project. Available at: http:// www.acgme.org/ outcome/comp/compFull.asp. Accessed May 2008.

5.   American Association of Colleges of Pharmacy. CAPE outcomes. Available at: http://www. aacp.org. Accessed May 2008.

6.   Bardes CL, Gillers D, Herman A. Learning to look: developing clinical observational skills at an art museum. *Med Educ*. 2001;35:1157–61.

7.   Purcell K. Pharmacy leadership survey: developing pharmacy leaders. *Texas Society of Health-System Pharmacists Journal*. 2001;27:10–4.

8.   Purcell K. Learning the skills and knowledge necessary to provide patient care. Texas Society of Health-System Pharmacists Newsletter. June 1996;25(4):8–9.

Tell me and I'll forget; show me and I may remember; involve me and I'll understand.
Chinese Proverb

Chapter 2

Necessary Skills for Effective Preceptors

Sara J. White, Diane B. Ginsburg, Lee C. Vermeulen, Stacy A. Taylor, Michael Piñón

Chapter Outline

Learning Objectives

- Define the elements of the communication process, and identify the preceptor's role in the communication process.
- List three interpersonal aspects of precepting.
- Describe three ways to be an effective clinical teacher.
- List at least three possible activities that will expose rotation students to leadership.

Effective preceptors need interpersonal skills in communication, teaching, and leadership. Sometimes the first step to becoming an effective preceptor is to assess your own skills as a pharmacist, communicator, educator, and mentor. Consider the following questions:

- How do I demonstrate to students the importance of cultivating the pharmacist-patient relationship?
- How do I respond to patient emotion, convey empathy, or motivate patients to change their behaviors?
- How do I use knowledge of the unique qualities of the patient, family, and community to improve outcomes?
- How do I provide timely and constructive feedback to my student?
- How can I manage time in a busy practice and balance my professional life?
- Am I encouraging postgraduate training?
- How can I give back or contribute to the profession?

These skills are rarely taught in pharmacy school so material outside of pharmacy becomes important to understand and apply.

Communication Skills

The ability to communicate well is one of the most important skills for practitioners in any situation. This is especially true for preceptors, as they must be able to communicate effectively with students to help them learn to be successful practitioners themselves.

The Communication Model

It is important for preceptors to understand how personal communication can affect their relationship with their students. To be an effective communicator (and hopefully an equally effective preceptor), an understanding of the basic communication model is important. The interpersonal communication model in Figure 2.1 is applicable to all situations, not just to pharmacy practice.

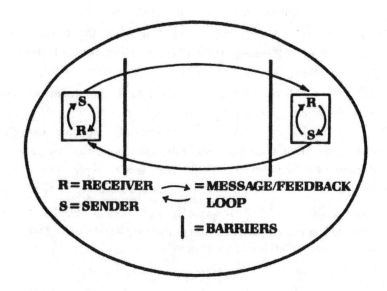

Figure 2.1. The interpersonal communication model (reproduced with permission from Beardsley RS, Kimberlin C, Tindall WN. *Communication Skills in Pharmacy Practice: A Practical Guide for Students and Practitioners.* 5th ed. Philadelphia, PA: Lippincott Williams & Wilkins; 2007).

The sender is the person who initiates the communication. This can occur in any setting: a face-to-face interaction, a phone call, an e-mail, or a text message. In a typical preceptor-student interaction, the preceptor acts as the sender when asking questions of a student—the receiver. The receiver is the person who receives the message and tries to decode it to determine what the sender is asking. The goal of communication is for the sender to deliver accurate information and for the receiver to understand the information presented.

Feedback occurs when the receiver and sender change roles in the communication process. This is the element of the communication model that makes communication a two-way process. In response to the message that the sender transmits, the receiver communicates back to the sender. This may occur in the form of an answer to a question or of an inquiry in response to a facial expression by the sender. Feedback can be both verbal and nonverbal. Sometimes a mere nodding of one's head can indicate to the sender that the receiver understands. In conversations involving a complex topic, feedback can be used to determine the level of understanding of the receiver. Feedback is a critical part of the communication process. When used effectively, this is where a sender can correct any miscommunication.

Barriers prevent effective communication and transmission of the message by preventing the receiver and sender from reading and decoding nonverbal communication. Barriers can be physical, such as counters or glass partitions; or they could be electronic, such as a phone call, e-mail, or text message. Removal of the physical barriers facilitates feedback and prevents miscommunication.

With electronic communication, such as e-mail messages, it is sometimes difficult to remove barriers, as the message must rely solely on the words contained in it. Word choice, or semantics, can indicate a tone that the sender of the message did not intend. Using all capital letters or no punctuation (often interpreted as "flaming" messages) can give the message a completely different meaning from what the sender intended. Without a webcam (which is only minimally effective to facilitate reading nonverbal communications), the only elements the receiver can decode are the words and phrasing of the message. To compound this, when the sender does not respond immediately to the receiver's response, the receiver may further read something negative in the message.

Effective communication ensures that students understand the information presented. When communication goes well, decoding the message is easy, but when the sender transmits one message verbally and another nonverbally, the receiver is unable to determine the sender's true message. Interpersonal communication is a fluid process. Verbal and nonverbal messages are being sent simultaneously and constantly between communicators. For example, you may say something complimentary to a student, but your nonverbal communication (e.g., facial expression, body language) may not support the verbal message. This is how miscommunication occurs.

The message is the most common place for miscommunication to occur. This is the element that is transmitted from one individual to another through various media (e.g., dialog or written communication). The manner in which the message is sent can change how others interpret and decode it. As with all aspects of the communication process, it is not only what you say, but also how you say it that can result in understanding or cause a breakdown in communication. As important as the actual words you select, nonverbal communication can support your message or cause miscommunication. It is very important that you remember that the student is decoding your nonverbal communication at the same time as the spoken message. Examples of nonverbal communication are as follows:

- Facial expressions
- Gestures
- Body language
- Posture
- Eye contact
- Tone of voice and inflection

In most situations, the sender formulates the message before it is transmitted, so if miscommunication occurs, it happens as a result of the method (i.e., wording or nonverbal communication) or media (e.g., dialog, e-mail, etc.) he or she uses to convey it. For example, a common communication mistake is to ask a closed-ended question while expecting a response to an open-ended question. The receiver may answer the yes/no question with *yes* or *no* instead of with the detailed response the sender expected. Simply by changing the beginning of the question (e.g., replacing "do you know" with "what is") will ask the correct question and will, in turn, elicit the expected response. You can easily create an open-ended question by beginning a question with who, what, when, where, why, or how.

• Preceptor Pearls •

Remember that how you say something is as important as what you say. Choose your words carefully and be aware of nonverbal communication.

Miscommunication is not limited to the interaction between preceptors and students. It can happen in all facets of life; however, this can be magnified during times of conflict and certainly when trying to teach students. It is easy for preceptors and students to become frustrated during experiential training when the objectives and outcomes for the rotation are not clearly stated. When this occurs, the expectations of the preceptor and student are not met, resulting in a negative learning experience. An example might be how many patients the student is expected to follow the medication therapy on.

Preceptors must be conscious of their communication style and manner in which they ask questions. Students coming out of pharmacy programs today are required to receive training in communication skills. Many preceptors did not have this type of course work or practical experiences as part of their curriculum. Questioning and listening skills are two areas that are covered in didactic courses through simulations and actual interactions with patients and other healthcare providers. Role-playing with observation and feedback from colleagues are two ways in which your questioning style can be evaluated.

• Preceptor Pearls •

Communication in any setting should be clear, concise, and fair.

Questioning and listening skills go hand-in-hand in effective communication. As discussed previously, the manner in which you ask a question can dictate the type of response (e.g., a closed-ended question typically results in a one-word response). All types of questions, including closed-ended, open-ended, leading, and probing questions, need to be incorporated in effective communication. Examples of these questions are shown in Box 2.1.

Box 2.1 • Types of Questions

Closed-ended	Have you ever prepared a TPN solution?
Open-ended	What are your goals for this rotation?
Leading	How would you counsel this patient?
Probing	What else could be done to minimize the side effect profile of the current regimen?

The key to getting the desired response is directly related to the type of question asked. This is important for preceptors and students as miscommunication can and will occur if one of the parties asks the wrong type of question for the expected type of answer. This is a great learning exercise for both parties involved when feedback is incorporated. When feedback is used effectively, either party—sender or receiver—can indicate a level of understanding and use additional questions to elicit the desired information. Good questioning skills take practice and the willingness and awareness of others to provide input.

Listening skills are as important to effective communication as the manner in which a question is asked. Since students will mirror the behaviors of their preceptors, listening is a very important skill to learn and to demonstrate to students. However, being a good listener is not as easy as it seems. Active listening, or listening with the intent to understand, takes focus and desire on the part of the listener. It is easy to be distracted from listening to what others have to say. Phones, PDAs, other interruptions, and stress may cause even the most conscientious listener to stop listening. Sometimes, we fall into the habit of "selective listening," where we do not engage and barely appear to be listening by nodding our heads and mumbling, "uh huh," "hmm," or "okay." Most people can see that a person responding in this manner is not truly listening. If a preceptor does this frequently to a student, it is likely that the student will cease to ask questions or to talk to the preceptor because he or she will feel that the preceptor is not listening or is disinterested. Further, selective listening can cause a practitioner to miss crucial information when talking to patients.

• Preceptor Pearls •

Active listening is an important aspect of communication.

It is very gratifying to be a good listener. We can all probably remember a patient who we helped because we took the time to listen. It is important to remember to listen more than to talk. As the ancient Greek philosopher Zeno once said, "The reason we have two ears and only one mouth is that we may hear more and speak less."[1]

Written Communication

As knowledge-based professionals, pharmacists depend on their ability to transfer information in order to care effectively for patients. While that transfer of knowledge most often takes place verbally, written communication skills are also essential. As noted in recent surveys, written skills are not only needed by pharmacy administrators and educators but, increasingly, are also needed as a prerequisite for successful pharmacy practice in all settings.[2,3] Preceptors must be prepared to provide students with training on effective and efficient writing.

The first step in effectively teaching writing skills as a preceptor is to recognize that students may not realize the importance of being good writers. Preceptors must emphasize the fact that clear, concise, and informative writing can demonstrate professionalism and competence. Likewise, lack of clarity of thought and expression will quickly compromise a pharmacist's credibility in the eyes of patients and other professionals.

You (and your students) must also accept the fact that being able to write well is a skill that must be learned, practiced, and improved. As a preceptor, you will transfer writing skills passively to your students as they read your written work and recognize the quality of your writing. You must also respond to your students' written documents. Your willingness and ability to provide constructive criticism, by editing rather than simply critiquing their work, will determine the impact you will have on their writing skills.

Pharmacists are expected to write in a wide variety of formats, and preceptors should provide students with exposure to each of the various types of documents common in their practice area. It is useful to contrast differences in style, tone, and even grammatical form required of various written documents. For example, a particular form of writing is used for written progress notes in patients' medical records that may not necessarily emphasize precise grammar, sentence structure, or even punctuation. In contrast, higher expectations are normally set for new drug monographs written for presentation to Pharmacy and Therapeutics Committees. However, accuracy of information, appropriate use of medical terminology, avoidance of dangerous abbreviations, and correct spelling are important issues regardless of the context.

Institution-specific style manuals should be developed and provided to students to assist in identifying important writing conventions relevant to particular types of written documents. In the absence of a particular desired format, the *American Medical Association Manual of Style* can serve as a guide for appropriate format, style, and tone of most technical biomedical writing (including issues such as appropriate citation format, technical terminology, and abbreviation standards).[4] Simply requiring students to read several examples of particular document types will assist them in adopting the appropriate tone and format. One of the most valuable tools for honing writing skills is Strunk and White's *The Elements of Style*.[5] The full text of the most recent edition (published in 1999) can also be accessed free online at http://www.bartleby.com/141. It is an in indispensable guide to good writing that should be read and reread before undertaking any substantial writing. Additionally, you should ensure that students have access to a standard collegiate dictionary, a medical dictionary, and a thesaurus for their use during clerkship rotations.

• Preceptor Pearls •

Strunk and White's *The Elements of Style* is an invaluable resource for improving writing skills.

Once students have completed a written document, the preceptor should edit it using a coaching approach. Rather than simply identifying an error or unclear phrase, sentence, or paragraph and expecting an appropriate change, suggest specific corrections or even offer completely rewritten alternative sentences in the margin. Writers improve when better writers edit their work. After students receive feedback in this way, they are better prepared to accurately and clearly articulate similar thoughts and information in the future. Therefore, editing serves two roles—to improve the writing of the moment and to improve future writing.

Preceptors may also need to assist students with particular writing challenges, such as overcoming writer's block or improving the writing of students who are not native-English speakers. A variety of writing resources are available at most colleges, and preceptors should familiarize themselves with those resources. A word of caution, however: many writing clinics guide liberal arts and general education students, and their staff is often unfamiliar with the technical conventions used in biomedical writing.

Finally, new preceptors working with students often find the opportunity to complete projects that are worthy of publication in peer-reviewed journals. Manuscript preparation is particularly challenging, but it can also be exceptionally rewarding for preceptors and students. Pharmacy faculty can often provide guidance, support, and assistance in that effort.

Development of good communications skills is an important component of the internship experience. Effective communication is vital for both the preceptor and the student. Adherence to the model for effective communication can prevent miscommunication from occurring. Students and preceptors should be mindful that communication is not just face-to-face interactions but encompasses all facets of communication (e.g., verbal, written, electronic, etc.). Care and nurture of the communication process can aide in facilitating a positive practice experience for all involved.

Interpersonal Skills to Benefit Preceptor and Student

As preceptors, students will look to you to gain from your wisdom and experiences in all aspects of performing your job. We generally think that experiential rotations provide an opportunity for students to begin applying their knowledge of the appropriate uses of medications, and for preceptors to serve as resources to augment and supplement this knowledge base. While this is true, our daily actions will also provide a model of how a pharmacist functions to fit into the overall healthcare environment. Demonstrating warmth, interest, and compassion in your relationships with your students and with patients will encourage your students to act the same way toward you and toward patients.

By observing and working alongside practicing pharmacists, students begin to develop their attitudes and abilities to interact with others. Therefore, it is important to continue to develop your skills of working with other healthcare professionals as you develop skills of interacting with the students you are precepting. A secondary benefit of forming strong relationships with colleagues and peers is the potential for greater career advancement and enhanced psychosocial support.[6]

• Preceptor Pearls •

Having good interpersonal skills not only demonstrates to students an appropriate way to act, but it can also provide you with personal and career benefits.

Students who are just beginning a new rotation are often nervous or intimidated about being placed in a patient care situation in which they lack confidence and experience. The first few moments of positive interaction between students and a preceptor can quickly begin to put the students at ease and will demonstrate that you are genuinely interested in the student. Students are more relaxed and ready to learn when they have a preceptor who is warm, friendly, enthusiastic, and pleasant. Students can easily perceive whether or not the preceptor is happy to have them and interested in their academic and personal needs.

As a preceptor, it is beneficial to develop professional friendships with your students and future colleagues. Students may have a variety of personal struggles outside of their professional life ranging from family illness to financial hardship. On the other hand, students may also struggle through a rotation due to lack of adequate sleep, preparation, or commitment to the rotation. When you have a good rapport with students you will often know the true reason for a particular student's tardiness or failure to complete an assignment and be able to provide an empathetic and appropriate response. An understanding and caring preceptor can offer encouragement to students facing difficult times or can attempt to motivate wayward students. Regardless of the situation, it is difficult to meet students' academic needs without first displaying a caring and compassionate attitude toward students as individuals.

It is often difficult to maintain confidence in your own knowledge base when students seem to know all the latest information on a particular medication or disease state. This can be especially challenging for young practitioners or for seasoned practitioners who are new at precepting. However, when interacting with students it is important to convey confidence in yourself, in the services you provide, and in your real-world experience. It is not necessary for you to be an expert on all subjects to be a successful preceptor. Be a lifelong learner and take the opportunity to learn new concepts from students; it will only strengthen the bond when students realize you are willing to listen and learn.

• Preceptor Pearls •

It is not necessary for you to be an expert on all subjects to be a successful preceptor. Be willing to listen to your students and learn something new.

It is important to develop healthy professional relationships with coworkers and members of various healthcare disciplines. The best way to form friendships is to be friendly, kind, and considerate. Make a conscious effort to smile and interact with people at work. Develop a genuine interest in others. Ask them questions about themselves, their families, and their hobbies. In a similar manner, it is important that you be willing to share information about yourself. It can also help your professional relationships to participate in workplace conversations. Your friendliness will make other people more comfortable coming to you with their medication-related questions or to ask your assistance on a drug-related topic that they just do not understand. Further, establishing and maintaining professional relationships will provide opportunities for networking.

Leaders who exhibit positive behaviors such as hope, confidence, and optimism obtain better outcome from others than leaders who do not.[7] It is important not only to communicate your expectations, but also to convey your confidence in the student's ability to achieve those expectations. Maintaining confidence in the abilities of yourself and your student will often cause students to work even harder to reach goals. Additionally, optimistic people tend to be more pleasant to be around. Be cognizant of the attitude you project and how this impacts your ability to get the most from your students.

Building trust takes time, but is a crucial element for any pharmacist who wants to significantly impact patient care. Once trust is established, others respect your judgment and know they can rely on you for credible information that can be directly applied without the need for excessive questioning. In order to build trust, you must demonstrate consistency in your actions. Always be honest, reliable, and predictable.[8] This means that you act in an honest and ethical manner, show up for work and meetings on time, provide accurate responses, follow up on pending issues, and meet deadlines. As you demonstrate your trustworthiness, other colleagues will begin to place more trust in you and your credibility will grow. When teaching students, remember to teach them that trust takes a long time to build, can be destroyed quickly, and is much more difficult to regain a second time around.

In developing integrity, it is important to first have a solid foundation of central beliefs and values by which you conduct your life. Daily decisions can then be made within the context of this value system. Trust and integrity go hand in hand; once integrity of character has been developed it is much easier to gain trust. People will come to rely on you to provide honest and consistent answers, backed up by sound reasoning and data, and that you will be accountable for your actions.

Be a Coach

Students rely on their preceptors to "coach" and provide feedback on their performance. A coach helps students focus on a specific aspect of behavior, performance, or life. While the focus is on learning and self-awareness, coaching helps the student find their own best answers to problem-solving. When students are developing new skills, it is important to concentrate on providing specific positive feedback for work well done.

Constructive feedback should be tailored to help students understand their learning needs. Feedback is most effective when it is descriptive of specific situations and skills and when it is given soon after the preceptor's observation of these events. Appropriate and timely feedback reinforces what has been done correctly, reviews what areas warrant improvement, and corrects mistakes. Coaching in this manner proves to be less judgmental than evaluation and is best given informally throughout the student's experience. In addition, if the student has the opportunity to self-assess prior to hearing the preceptor's comments, the feedback provided is typically more meaningful.

Self-assessment questions provide opportunities for the student to share his or her approach or rationale while allowing for constructive and engaging discussion. Questions might include the following:

- "What were the major findings that led to your conclusion?"
- "What else needs to be considered?"
- "What are the key features of this case?"
- "What are the next steps?"
- "What are your thoughts about how you addressed this patient's questions about their drug regimen?"
- "How would you have improved or done this differently?"

Students should understand that their rotation is an environment in which they will learn by experience and inquiry. This will allow them to comfortably disclose uncertainties or learning needs.

As you assume your role as a preceptor, remember the importance of developing good interpersonal skills. Students will be observing you as a role model for how a pharmacist interacts with other members of the healthcare world. Developing excellent interpersonal skills will also help you in precepting students, making them feel more at ease and comfortable in the learning environment.

Teaching Skills

Today's students respond well in an active learning environment. They need to strive to apply or put into practice the information they are learning. For example, a preceptor can explain the important aspects of sterile technique; however, unless the student actually compounds a sterile parenteral solution, they will probably not develop the critical skills necessary to learn this technique. The majority of training students have had prior to starting their Advanced Practice Pharmacy Experiences (APPEs) has been in didactic lectures and simulations. Although students have been exposed to clinical practice through Introductory Pharmacy Practice Experiences (IPPEs), their hands-on participation may be limited depending on the program and rotation experience.

• Preceptor Pearls •

Providing students with opportunities to practice their skills will help them better retain the information.

Many pharmacists who decide to teach students do so with little formal training in teaching and instructional design. Although some preceptors may have been exposed to and/or involved in organized teaching during their training (Pharm.D. curriculum and/or residency), the majority of preceptors do not have a background in teaching methods and learning styles. Most preceptors are very good at communicating clinical information, but the students they are precepting sometimes have difficulty applying this clinical information because of the manner in which their preceptors present the information. The pharmacist who is a great clinician is not necessarily the best teacher and vice versa.

What can preceptors do to be better teachers? The following are some helpful hints to being an effective clinical teacher[9]:

1. A model of desired performance helps students. Positive examples of what to do are more effective than what not to do.
2. Provide verbal cues that identify key features of the skill.
3. Simplified and step-wise instructions are best.
4. Permit students the maximum freedom to experience successful completion of a task. This will facilitate their knowledge and skill development.
5. Provide positive and constructive feedback.
6. Don't try to correct everything on the first attempt. The best way for a student to learn is sometimes by failing.
7. High-level skills are developed through much practice.
8. As you evaluate work, verbalize the process you are using and the basis for your evaluation.

Reflect on your own experiences and incorporate them into your teaching styles. Did you have a great professor and/or preceptor who you really admired while you were a student? These are the individuals you want to emulate. Excellent preceptors possess the following qualities[10]:

- They are supportive of and respectful to their students, colleagues, and patients.
- They are excellent role models and look for opportunities to demonstrate excellence in practice.
- They exude enthusiasm for their practice, their patients, and for teaching students.

There are many ways that preceptors can improve their teaching skills. Having a true desire to teach and to give back to the profession is the most important criterion. Many schools offer or require specific preceptor continuing education and training. Frequently, these types of workshops and programs cover everything from teaching skills to assessment.

Leadership Skills

Teaching leadership skills and identifying potential leaders is critical for pharmacy's future. In 2005, White documented that by 2015 approximately 80% of the current health-system directors of pharmacy do not anticipate being in their current positions. Since there are around 5,800 hospitals, this will present a need of more than 4,000 new directors. Likewise about 77% of the pharmacy middle managers (associate directors, assistant directors, supervisors, clinical coordinators, etc.) indicated they would not be functioning as middle managers in 10 years. The survey respondents indicated the main reason for this turnover is attrition through retirement. Looking at the potential leadership interest in the current practitioners this study found that only 30% would be interested in moving into a leadership position sometime in their career, while 62% of the pharmacy students surveyed indicated an interest. In addition to the need for directors, a significant need will exist for current practitioners to move into this middle management leadership role.[11]

With a large number of leadership positions becoming vacant and very few current practitioners interested in filling them, there is a significant risk that especially the director of pharmacy position may be filled by a nonpharmacist such as a nurse, a materials manager, a physician, an MHA (masters in health administration), an MBA (masters in business administration), etc. Health-system organizations may have no choice as they need to have pharmacy leadership and a pharmacist can be the Board of Pharmacy Pharmacist in Charge without being the director of pharmacy. It is more beneficial to the site for a pharmacist to act as the director, and nonpharmacists could perform some of the middle management roles such as financial management or human resources, under the guidance of a pharmacist director.

To ensure pharmacist leadership into the future, we need both Big L pharmacist and Little L pharmacist leaders. The Big L leaders are those with a formal title such as chief pharmacy officer, director, associate director, assistant director, supervisor, clinical coordinator, etc., whereas the Little L leaders include every pharmacist on his or her shift in the practice.

• Preceptor Pearls •

Both Big L and Little L leaders are critical to the advancement of the pharmacy profession.

Leadership is crucial because it helps the advancement of the profession in immeasurable ways. Before the 1960s, pharmacists did not typically practice in hospitals, and the rare hospital pharmacy was generally in the basement. Nurses prepared intravenous admixtures and took the oral doses they needed from stock bottles on their unit, rather than relying on hospital pharmacists. Clinical pharmacy services as we now know them began in the late 1960s when pharmacists left the basement pharmacies to participate in medical rounds and to better utilize their therapeutic expertise to make prescribing and medication monitoring decisions. Each of these service innovations resulted not just from Big L leaders but also from many Little L leaders taking calculated risks, setting up the services, and performing the day-to-day activities. This evolution of pharmacy services is one example of how important pharmacist leadership is to the profession.

It is paramount that every preceptor incorporates leadership exposure and training into rotations, even the purely clinical rotations. Leadership and clinical practice are integrated skills for every pharmacist as a Little L leader so that practice continues to evolve. The preceptor's goal must be to build every future pharmacist's leadership confidence so he or she will continue evolving services. The preceptor is the role model that the student and resident emulate so it is important that the preceptor believe in this integration of leadership and clinical practice. Consider the benefits your Little L leadership in practice has created both for your patients and for your career.

To understand leadership it is helpful to contrast it with management. Management is what all pharmacists do very well in processing their work. A manager focuses on maintaining the system and ensuring that things are done correctly, and relies on checks as controls. Managers maintain the status quo and focus on the short term. Stated another way, the ASHP Required and Elective Educational Outcomes, Goals, Objectives, and Instructional Objectives for Postgraduate Year One (PGY1) Pharmacy Practice Residency Glossary defines management practices as planning, organizing, implementing, and monitoring and evaluating.[12] Specific examples appear below. See Box 2.2.

Box 2.2 • The Precepting Leadership Continuum

Leadership Exposure Activities

- Provide messages to students (repeat frequently; once is not enough)
  - Remind them that every pharmacist is a Little L leader during a shift or in his or her practice
  - Share your personal experience of how pharmacy services have improved during your career and what future trends might be
  - Describe what leadership means (both Big L and Little L)
- Encourage students to attend meetings (committee/staff/faculty) with you; their focus should be on the following:
  - Interactions among caregivers (both effective and ineffective)
  - Pharmacist input and impact
  - How to productively function in a meeting
- Help them arrange to shadow/observe Big L Leaders and focus on
  - What leaders do, who they interact with, what they are trying to achieve
  - How their career has evolved
  - Their impact (actual and potential)
- Suggest they do small actual projects (e.g., performance improvement, formulary, data analysis) that include making recommendations for changes

Box 2.2 • The Precepting Leadership Continuum (cont'd)

- Recommend professional organizational leadership opportunities
  - Attend meetings/committees/Board of Director/interview elected officers
  - Set them up for student/new practitioner involvement opportunities/push news/list serves
- Suggest they read Stephen Covey's *The 7 Habits of Highly Effective People* (in the self-development section of any bookstore)

Identify Potential Big L Leaders

- Look for characteristics that enable people to be effective leaders; some have the following qualities:
  - Are passionate about what they do and are willing to work hard
  - Are good with people, get along with everyone, have concern for others, and share credit
  - Are reasonably organized and confident
  - Have good verbal communication skills
  - Make decisions, use good judgment, and take responsibility
  - Think broadly, beyond the pharmacy task at hand; are curious; ask questions; and identify service problems and propose solutions
- Frequently convey the following messages to students
  - Remind them that they have leadership skills; use specific examples and affirm what they do well because frequently they are unaware of their strengths
  - Suggest that they take on projects beyond just doing the requirements. By doing so, they will learn to work efficiently and to balance competing priorities, two skills they will need in their practice.
  - Encourage them to consider some time in their career taking a formal leadership position
  - Encourage them to think, question the status quo, and propose changes. Reinforce when they do, no matter how small an effort they make.

Leadership Training: Make Additional Opportunities Available

- Messages for students
  - Suggest that they find a Big L leader mentor. Have them formally ask someone they are comfortable with to help them with their careers. Spend time asking them for advice.
  - Help them learn by observing other successful people so that they can see what works and what does not work

Box 2.2 • The Precepting Leadership Continuum (cont'd)

- Stress the importance of learning from your own experiences. Tell them to ask for feedback on ideas and approach.

- Suggest they investigate Health-System Administration Accredited Residencies through the ASHP website. Even if they are not interested in a residency now, they may be in the future.

- Suggest they research practitioner leadership training opportunities through the ACCP and ASHP Foundation websites in case they are interested once they move into practice.

• Expand leader shadowing/observations; include different types, if possible, such as residency program directors, school department chairs, or others outside of pharmacy

• Actual projects

• Challenge them with "what if" leadership scenarios that do not have one right answer

• Attend pharmacy leadership team meetings

• Report on meetings attended, content, and human dynamics

• Suggest possible readings

- Bush PW, Walesh SG. *Managing & Leading 44 Lessons Learned for Pharmacists.* Bethesda, MD: ASHP; 2008.

- Leadership book summaries: Available at http://www.summaries.com

- Leadership abstracts: Available at http://www.getabstract.com

- Leadership books written by John Maxwell, Ken Blanchard, or Spencer Johnson, all of which can be found in any bookstore in the business section

Leadership, on the other hand, involves identifying the right things to do and inspiring others through a compelling vision. Leaders make people feel significant and develop a sense of commitment that fosters teamwork that, in turn, excites people through their own enthusiasm and passion. Leaders challenge the status quo and try new ways of organizing and processing work; they are innovators. Leaders take calculated risks, making adjustments as they gain experience. They have a bias for action or getting things done and hold themselves responsible and accountable. The ASHP Required and Elective Educational Outcomes, Goals, Objectives, and Instructional Objectives for Postgraduate Year One (PGY1) Pharmacy Practice Residency Glossary defines leadership as scanning, focusing, aligning/mobilizing, and inspiring.[12] Specific examples are contained in Box 2.2. Simply put, leaders are change agents who use their creative dissatisfaction with the status quo to innovate and improve services. Every pharmacist has an impact and with some leadership skills the legacy they leave can maximize their potential.

Think of precepting leadership as a continuum beginning with exposure, continuing through identifying potential leaders, and as time permits, leadership training. Refer to Box 2.2 for the continuum from exposure through actual leadership training. Suggestions for each point on the continuum appear in Box 2.2. The preceptor needs to provide the suggested messages so the student puts this leadership involvement in the proper context and realizes its future application to his or her practice. The preceptor must be interested in the students as individuals and provide time to listen to their experiences. As a preceptor helps the student develop his or her leadership skills, the teacher-student relationship develops more into one between colleagues. This evolution provides students with the expectation that they begin to perform more as a pharmacist than as a student. Devoting time to the student and the leadership activities nurtures his or her leadership involvement, which is, in turn, making an investment in the future of the profession.

• Preceptor Pearls •

Leadership activities expose students to leadership and teach them to become leaders on their own.

No matter what leadership activity the students perform, preceptors must set them up for success to help build their confidence. Clearly describe what to expect with the activity, why it is important, and what to look for as a learning experience. Express your confidence in them and set up a time to "debrief" after the activity by having them share their experiences. Ask questions that challenge them on what they learned and how they might apply it in their practice. Then set up another activity and repeat the process as time permits.

Precepting Leadership in Residencies

Leadership training is integral in pharmacy practice residencies and should build upon the individual resident's leadership exposure from their clerkships. Remember that residency program directors serve as leaders. The ASHP Accreditation Standard for Postgraduate Year One (PGY1) Pharmacy Residency Programs defines as one purpose "to further the development of leadership skills that can be applied in any position and in any practice setting."[13] The residency standards go on to say that "specifically residents will be held responsible and accountable for acquiring these outcome competencies…exercising leadership and practice management."[13] The ASHP accreditation Educational Goals and Objectives list the following as leadership goals[13]:

- R3.1 Exhibit essential personal skills of a practice leader.
- R3.2 Contribute to departmental leadership and management activities.
- R3.3 Exercise practice leadership.
- R4.0 Demonstrate project management skills.

Each of these goals has suggested ways to achieve the goals. The ASHP Section of Pharmacy Practice Managers compiled a list of ways preceptors were meeting these goals.[14] ASHP has a PGY2 residency accreditation standard in Health-System Pharmacy Administration, which has specific goals and objectives and can be found on the accreditation website.[15]

Preceptors are critical to providing leadership experience for all future pharmacists and ensuring that pharmacy services will continue to evolve in support of optimum patient care.

References

1. Wilkin NE. *Handbook for Pharmacy Educators: Contemporary Teaching Principles and Strategies.* Binghamptom, NY: Pharmaceutical Products Press; 2000.

2. Hobson EH, Waite NM, Briceland LL. Writing tasks performed by doctor of pharmacy students during clerkship rotations. *Am J Health Syst Pharm.* 2002;59:58–62.

3. Kennicutt JD, Hobson EH, Briceland LL, et al. On-the-job writing tasks of clerkship preceptors. *Am J Health Syst Pharm.* 2002;59:63–7.

4. Iverson C, et al, ed. *American Medical Association Manual of Style. 10th ed.* New York, NY: Oxford University Press; 2007.

5. Strunk W, White EB. *The Elements of Style. 4th ed.* Neeham Heights, MA: Allyn and Bacon; 2000. Available at http://www.bartleby.com/141/. Accessed June 3, 2008.

6. Hitchcock MA, Bland CJ, Hekelman FD, et al. Professional networks: the influence of colleagues on the academic success of faculty. *Acad Med.* 1995;70:1108–16.

7. Gardner WL, Schermerhorn JR. *Organizational Dynamics.* 2004;33(3):270–81.

8. Robbins SP. *The Truth About Managing People.* Upper Saddle River, NJ: Prentice Hall; 2003.

9. McKeachie WJ. *Teaching Tips: A Guidebook for the Beginning College Teacher.* Lexington, MA: DC Heath and Company; 1986:135–6.

10. Paulman PM, Susman JL, Abboud CA. *Precepting Medical Students in the Office.* Baltimore, MD: The Johns Hopkins University Press; 2000:70–1.

11. White S. Will there be a pharmacy leadership crisis? An ASHP foundation scholar-in-residence report. *Am J Health Syst Pharm.* 2005;62:845–55.

12. The ASHP Required and Elective Educational Outcomes, Goals, Objectives, and Instructional Objectives for Postgraduate Year One (PGY1) Pharmacy Residency Programs. Available at: http://www.ashp.org/S_ASHP/docs/files/RTP_PGY1GoalsObjectives.doc. Accessed April 2008.

13. ASHP Accreditation Standard for Postgraduate Year One (PGY1) Pharmacy Residency Programs. Available at: http://www.ashp.org/S_ASHP/docs/files/RTP_PGY1Accredstandard.pdf. Accessed April 2008.

14. Pharmacy Practice Residency (PGY1) Pharmacy Residency Helpful Ideas for Activities to Provide Leadership Training. Available at: http://www.ashp.org/S_ASHP/docs/files/ResidencyLeadershipTraining.pdf. Accessed April 2008.

15. Educational Outcomes, Goals, and Objectives for Postgraduate Year Two (PGY2) Health-System Pharmacy Administration Residency Program. Available at: http://www.ashp.org/S_ASHP/docs/files/RTP_objhealth sysphadministration032608.doc. Accessed April 2008.

Suggested Readings

Jastrzembski J. New practitioner forum developing leadership skills. *Am J Health Syst Pharm.* 2007;64:1900–3.

Maxwell JC. *Developing the Leaders Around You.* Nashville, TN: Thomas Nelson; 1995.

Pierpaoli PG, Flint NB. Residency training—the profession's forge for leader development. *Pharm Pract Manag Q.* 1995;2:44–56.

Zellmer WA. Doing what needs to be done in pharmacy practice leadership: a message to residents. *Am J Health Syst Pharm.* 2003;60:1903–7.

Zellmer WA. Reason and history as guides for pharmacy practice leaders. *Am J Health Syst Pharm.* 2005;62:838–44.

By learning you will teach, by teaching you will learn.
Latin proverb

Chapter 3

Preceptor-Student Relationship

Dana S. Fitzsimmons, James Colbert, Jr., Roy T. Hendley, Grace M. Kuo, Andrew Laegeler, Jennifer L. Ridings-Myhra

Chapter Outline

Learning Objectives

- Define and discuss an effective preceptor-student relationship from both a student's and preceptor's perspective.
- Describe the desired characteristics of a proficient preceptor from the student's view.
- Outline the roles, responsibilities, expectations, and goals of preceptors and students during pharmacy practice experiences.
- Utilize motivational theory to encourage performance and engage students in successful experiential rotations.
- Identify steps that can be taken to provide an optimal setting to ensure a positive experience for all involved including interns, preceptors, and the sites.

There are many things that contribute to a successful student practical experience. One of the most important contributing factors is the development of a positive student-preceptor relationship. Identifying ways to foster that relationship from student and preceptor perspectives will help. Understanding expectations, roles, responsibilities and identifying goals sets the foundation for success. The preceptor can further enhance the likelihood of a great experience by utilizing motivational theory and by structuring a positive learning environment. This chapter focuses on the relationship and creating an environment where that relationship can flourish.

Establishing an Effective Preceptor-Student Relationship: The Preceptor's Perspective

The Preceptor's Professional Characteristics

Effective preceptors have certain characteristics in common. They are enthusiastic, energetic, knowledgeable, self-confident, work well under stress, and are willing to learn. They enjoy their work, freely share information, and seek to further develop their professional skills. They also enjoy teaching and learning from their students. Aware of their duties as professional role models, preceptors inspire students to develop their professional skills and show students how to establish professional relationships.

The Preceptor's Teaching Style

Anthony Grasha has identified five different teaching styles—expert, formal authority, personal model, facilitator, and delegator—that can be combined in various ways to achieve effective teaching.[1] Similarly, Neal Whitman described two learning styles that could be applied to the practice setting—pedagogy (teacher-centered) and andragogy (learner-centered).[2] Because experiential rotations are especially designed for students to develop hands-on clinical skills, experiential teaching is more learner-centered and requires the preceptor to be a model and a facilitator.

A Chinese proverb says "Tell me and I forget. Show me and I remember. Involve me and I understand." A good preceptor demonstrates for the students and involves students in the process of learning. Guiding students to apply their knowledge into practice by having open discussions and competency evaluations facilitates more effective learning for students in the practice setting. Designating specific times weekly for the purpose of reflection can also be helpful. Reflection is a time when the preceptor and students can discuss student feelings of security or insecurity in learning and/or ways of coping with mental stress during the rotation.

The Preceptor's Interaction with Students

To establish a dynamic relationship with students, the preceptor must be willing to invest the time and effort needed to communicate effectively with students. Effective communication requires that the preceptor be sensitive to students' learning needs and be able to evaluate students' strengths and weaknesses without intimidation. Communication is a process, and different communication styles may be needed during the 4- or 6-week clerkship rotation. Initially, the preceptor may facilitate student learning by giving direct instruction. Gradually, as students become more familiar with the practice setting and more confident in their professional skills, the preceptor could assume the role of a coach, encouraging students to become more actively involved in the clinical practice. Appropriate feedback to students about their performance is essential, especially when preceptors discuss the goals/objectives and the performance expectations of the rotation with students. Preceptors also need to listen to and answer students' questions. Continual open communication will encourage students to keep asking questions and will help them solve problems and make decisions. (Refer to Chapter 2 for more discussion on establishing good communication.)

• Preceptor Pearls •

Understand your role in the preceptor-student relationship: as a mentor, facilitator, and role model to students. Remember that the intern's role is still that of a student and not an employee.

A supportive preceptor concentrates his or her energy on bringing out the best potential in trainees. The preceptor communicates clearly about learning objectives and goals; designs interactive learning activities; explains and shares professional information and personal experience; demonstrates skills; provides timely feedback; and encourages continual learning despite failures and imperfections. Though training may involve diligent discipline and growing pains, the preceptor guides student trainees during the difficult stages of the learning process and delights in seeing students become better practitioners. By having respect for their students, preceptors can foster meaningful and lasting professional relationships.

Establishing an Effective Preceptor-Student Relationship: The Recent Graduate's Perspective

Current and future pharmacy preceptors, do you remember when you were a pharmacy student? Maybe it was last year or maybe it was many years ago. No matter how long ago it was, you can probably remember a few influential moments you had during your years as a student. It's likely that those moments were associated with an individual whom you connected with and who encouraged you to achieve more than you thought possible. Those rewarding experiences were with other people because connecting with people was the initial reason to get into pharmacy practice.

Before you had a great pharmacy practice experience, you likely began to forge a strong professional relationship with a pharmacist. Some interpersonal relationships happen with very little effort. Two people just "click." At other times, it may appear that there is no chance of a relationship. The preceptor and student agree to peacefully coexist until their time together is over. Leaving a relationship to "chance" puts the preceptor, the student, and the experience in danger before the rotation even begins.

A contentious preceptor-student relationship will almost certainly frustrate both the preceptor and student. The learning experience might be blunted. The student may feel short-changed by the rotation experience and may not appreciate the preceptor's knowledge, skills and abilities. The preceptor may have feelings of guilt and wonder "What just happened?" Conversely, a cooperative preceptor-student relationship will be one where both the preceptor and student look forward to working together. They will jointly seek out opportunities to advance the learning experience. The preceptor may learn from the student, who is up-to-date and current with the school's pharmacy curriculum. The student will appreciate the preceptor's practical experience and knowledge. Before either person knows it, they will have formed a bond that will last for years. Those preceptors will be the ones that the students recall inspiring them to be the pharmacist they are today.

Do good preceptor-student relationships just happen? Or, can every preceptor-student relationship be a good one? If the preceptor invests the time and effort, and puts the student at the center of the learning experience, every preceptor-student relationship can be effective and rewarding for both parties. Placing the student's needs at the center of the experience is the most important paradigm. Many preceptors expect students to understand them, what is going on in their lives and careers. However, most students are in their mid-twenties, and while interested and devoted to their new pharmacy career, they are still trying to discover themselves. Recognizing this fact, remembering your own experiences at this age, and putting the student first will frame the preceptor-student relationship for a mutually positive experience.

The student arrives at a rotation site with work-related needs and expectations. Multiple organizational behavior theorists have described these needs as existing in a hierarchy or perhaps as lower order and higher order needs. These lower order needs must be met to allow fulfillment of higher order activities and accomplishments. These needs are a useful starting point to begin a discussion of how to better relate to students. Here are some of my suggestions in addressing student needs:

- Promptly provide some basic information about the site to the student. Where can they obtain food and beverage? What hours and schedules are expected of the student? What parking options are available to the student? Are there safety concerns that the student should be aware of?

- Provide a safe and positive learning environment. Select employees and coworkers for interaction with the student carefully as important impressions and aspirations are being formed by the student.

- Make the student feel important. The student is the center and focus of the rotation from their perspective and you can make the student sense that by being knowledgeable of their prior rotation experience and by discussing it with the student. Show a sincere interest in the student and in their career and personal goals.

- Establish clear goals and expectations. Review the goals frequently, be organized, be consistent and be reliable. Have a plan but remain flexible.

- Teach the student and build the student's self esteem. Respect the student as an individual. Be a guide or a coach as the student discovers new practice areas and synthesizes prior learning experiences. When a preceptor-student relationship reaches this level, it is the opportunity for greatest growth. The preceptor and student continually challenge each other to provide a renewing environment of learning. All preceptor-student relationships can reach this level.

• Preceptor Pearls •

Be sure to carefully select coworkers who will interact with the students. Bad first impressions and poor employee attitudes can negatively impact the student's experience.

Finally, preceptors who involve themselves professionally in students' lives, and who involve students in their lives, will have the greatest impact and the most rewarding preceptor-student relationships. However, preceptors cannot put their career objectives, day-to-day responsibilities or family life on hold in order to provide this student-centered experience. The key is to have an open dialogue. Communicate personal expectations, goals, outside commitments, and feedback on performance to students. No one aspect is more important than another. Students will learn that successful preceptors are people too in order to develop into successful preceptors themselves. Appreciating the student as a whole person and communicating with them on a peer level demonstrates leadership, commitment and compassion. Learning will flourish in such a relationship.

Students often use preceptors for letters of recommendation for jobs and residencies. In this setting, the student is using the preceptor to influence others and preceptors can provide great assistance. In addition, if the preceptor makes the student the center of the experience and truly develops the student, the preceptor can use the student as a reference for his/her work. That letter will read "Look at this student I precepted and how much he/she achieved. We had a great relationship and the student will be a high performer for you, too." Congratulations to that preceptor for achieving an effective preceptor-student relationship. Let's ensure that every student has that relationship and that the outcome is a great experience for everyone!

Student Expectations of a Proficient Preceptor

Experiential rotations are supervised practice opportunities which allow student pharmacists to observe and actively incorporate didactic knowledge to advanced pharmacy concepts for the improvement of the delivery of healthcare. Practicing preceptors in a variety of settings are exceptionally qualified to facilitate the development of student pharmacists in this advanced practice role. Because each student pharmacist enters the rotation with a varied amount of past experience and technical competence, providing learning opportunities which support the student's individual learning needs may be challenging.

Students have enormous expectations of experiential learning when entering their rotations. Their expectations are a product of 3–5 years of structured didactic learning. Students thirst for guided learning opportunities from preceptors to correlate textbook with clinical practice knowledge. They anticipate preceptors to provide opportunities to build on their drug knowledge from didactic coursework and prior rotations. The transition to experiential rotations provokes student anxiety as they learn to apply knowledge and validate competency prior to graduation. These expectations and their eagerness to display proficiency may be unrealistic due to lack of practice setting and clinical experience and may cause students to be disappointed with rotational experiences. Ultimately, students on rotation want a contributory role, an opportunity to apply and offer evidence-based recommendations, and the chance to mature as competent practitioners. As a result, students have significant expectations of their preceptors.

Preceptors supervise, mentor, and promote the professional development of student pharmacists. The preceptor's role is to facilitate the professional development of a student pharmacist throughout the rotation to allow the student to build on prior knowledge. The Academic-Practice Partnership Initiative of the American Association of Colleges of Pharmacy created a list of criteria for excellence of preceptors. The criteria include the following skills and attributes as essential components of being an effective and successful preceptor.

The preceptor should

1. possess leadership/management skills,

2. embody his/her practice philosophy,

3. be a role-model practitioner,

4. be an effective, organized, and enthusiastic teacher,

5. encourage self-directed learning of the student with constructive feedback and

6. have well-developed interpersonal/communication skills.[3]

The section in Chapter 1 entitled "Integrating Pharmacy Students into Your Practice" provides detailed instructions for preceptors on incorporating students into a rotation. Students expect that preceptors are prepared and eager to teach with the appreciation for different learning styles. A student knowledge level and experience to date assessment should be conducted by the preceptor to help modify and develop individualized and specific learning topics, goals, and objectives for the student's rotation. Performing a gap analysis enables the preceptor to avoid repeating material that the student may have mastered and allows weaknesses in student knowledge/skills to be identified. Orientation is the ideal place to perform a gap analysis.[4] Furthering a student pharmacist's knowledge can be accomplished by incorporating and emphasizing the following: orientation, feedback and evaluation, and role modeling.

• Preceptor Pearls •

Don't wait until later in the rotation, utilize the orientation period as an opportune time to perform gap analysis.

Orientation

A comprehensive orientation is essential for building an effective learning experience and preparing your student pharmacist for success.[5] Devoting adequate orientation time empowers the student pharmacist to feel comfortable and participate in patient care and it creates a positive learning environment. Providing pertinent information at the *beginning* of the rotation is an effective mechanism in teaching students where to retrieve answers to their questions on the requirements of the rotation as well as eliminating the potential for unclear expectations. Precise goals and objectives should be developed, representing an agreement between preceptor and student of the responsibilities required for successful completion of the rotation. Preceptors should also provide documentation of their current job responsibilities along with contact information, and, if possible, a work schedule. All of this orientation work sets the stage for success.[6]

Feedback and Evaluation

Feedback and evaluation are essential for learning, improving performance, reinforcing appropriate behavior, correcting deficiencies, and promoting confidence. Feedback and evaluation are critical to ensure that objectives and goals are accomplished. Feedback has been described as information concerning a student's performance in a given activity that is intended to guide their future performance in that same or in a related activity.[7] Students expect feedback to be verbal, frequent or continual, constructive, preceptor specific, and used to assess objective achievement. In contrast, evaluation is a formal written summation based on student specific goals used for grading and assessing global performance. This evaluation should encompass the student's daily performance feedback and an assessment of fulfillment of their rotation goals. This correlation provides the student with a realistic expectation of their upcoming evaluation(s) and experiential rotation performance. Students should not be surprised by their final evaluation. Preceptors that place high importance on feedback and evaluation are able to provide an accurate and constructive evaluation of the student's experiential performance.

Role Modeling

Students expect that preceptors will adhere to the same standards and performance behaviors set forth for the students. Positive role modeling via professional socialization is considered the most important concept of improving professionalism among students.[8] Professional socialization is the process by which students learn and adopt the values, attitudes, and practice behaviors of a profession. This "hidden curricula" is largely influenced by the preceptor-student relationship during experiential rotations. It is essential that the preceptor act according to the American Pharmacists Association Code of Ethics for Pharmacists to influence students in a positive manner for the benefit of other healthcare professionals, patients, and the practice of pharmacy.[9] Students admire their preceptors and are eager to find mentors that emulate their career interests. This type of positive relationship builds an attitude that creates success beyond the experiential learning environment.

Summary

Precepting student pharmacists can often be a rewarding experience but requires adequate preparation. Preceptors should design and plan the students' rotation learning activities carefully in conjunction with his/her practice interests and goals. Frequent, timely, and specific feedback is essential for a student to improve practice skills. Students' capacity to incorporate didactic learning with practice skills depends to a great deal on the relationship with the preceptor. Preceptors have an enormous opportunity to develop and shape future pharmacists. This is a valuable service for student pharmacists, the profession of pharmacy and for the public's health.

Roles, Responsibilities, Expectations, and Goals of Preceptors and Students

As we've discussed throughout this chapter, the preceptor-student relationship can be a rewarding professional experience for both parties. The experience can in the best of situations provide memories that both the preceptor and student can carry with them throughout their respective careers. Of course, experiences will vary, but understanding the factors that contribute to a positive relationship between students and preceptors will go a long way to creating those positive memories and professional rewards. Although these factors are many and varied, in this section we want to examine those over which the "players"—student, preceptor, facility, college or school of pharmacy, and accrediting and licensing agencies—have some degree of influence. Within any given internship experience and focusing specifically on the preceptor-student interaction, these factors include the following.

Determining Roles

This is an important first step in establishing an effective teaching-learning relationship. It must be clearly understood by both preceptors and students well before the students arrive. The relationship is further advanced when both are comfortable in their roles. Over time and with experience, preceptors move more freely within their role, while students as novices in each new practice site may not be quite so comfortable, but should exhibit some degree of growth in knowledge, skills and professional maturity over the continuum of pharmacy practice experiences.

The role of the preceptor is multifaceted. He or she is a teacher, role model, supervisor, evaluator, and mentor to each assigned student. This means that the preceptor must be adaptable to each student with whom the preceptor comes in contact (in terms of the student's educational background, previous pharmacy practice experience, professional aspirations, personality and cultural background). Additionally, the preceptor was chosen for this role because, among other factors, the preceptor is a competent practitioner. Certainly, the 2007 ACPE Standards and Guidelines are clear in their expectations for preceptors, stating in Appendix C that preceptors should be "positive role models for students." Among a preceptor's desirable traits are that the preceptor is competent to practice in his or her position, practices ethically and with compassion, engages in continuing professional development, and desires to educate others, including students and residents, among other qualities.[10]

• Preceptor Pearls •

Preceptors must remember the influence and impact of their behavior and role model appropriately.

Precepting can be one of the most rewarding professional experiences in which a practitioner engages, but as a part of a larger array of professional responsibilities, it can also be one of the most challenging. Students must clearly understand their role as learners and developing professionals. In most pharmacy curricula, the preceptor-student relationship within the context of the internship constitutes the entire final year of the program as well as an array of experiences in the preceding P1–P3 years. Therefore, both students and preceptors should recognize that teaching and learning are ongoing during all years of the professional curriculum.

Students must exhibit and hone professional behaviors during the internship. Hopefully, they have been exposed to professional expectations early in the pharmacy program. Practice experiences over the course of the pharmacy curriculum should challenge students to apply and refine these behaviors. Students should, in essence, "look like" a pharmacist and a professional by the end of their experiential program. Some students will approach the role of learner and blossoming professional enthusiastically, while others will exhibit fear and trepidation, especially in introductory practice experiences. It can be an exhilarating time for students as they "try on" different areas of practice while moving closer to achieving their educational and professional goals. It can also be a sobering time as students recognize that they have so much more to learn.

Setting Mutual Goals

The success of the preceptor-student relationship is dependent on creating a "win-win" scenario for all of the players. Everyone involved must, therefore, work together to develop mutually agreeable goals. These goals should be realistic (is the student a P1 or P4?), measurable via some form of assessment (evaluation form or exam, for example) and mapped against educational outcomes, attainable (in the amount of time allotted for the practice experience and commensurate with the particular practice experience and environment), and timely. They can be short-term or long-term.

One mutual goal is the development of competent practitioners through the continuum of practice experiences. How is this carried out for the mutual benefit of all? For preceptors, it is the personally rewarding experience of assisting the profession's future by educating and training the pharmacy practitioners of tomorrow—this can be both a short-term and a long-term goal. For students, it is the fulfillment of educational goals, development of the knowledge, skills, attitudes and values necessary to enter the profession, and exposure to various careers in pharmacy. The practice facility may view hosting students as a way to preview future employees and recruit students to that particular site—a short-term goal with long-term implications. The college or school of pharmacy is able to utilize the talents of enthusiastic, motivated pharmacists and their innovative practices as part of the educational process. The roles and responsibilities of each of the players will differ, but the result is the same—a rewarding personal and professional endeavor and the advancement of the profession.

Defining Responsibilities

It is critical for preceptors and students to be aware of their part in the continuum of curricular-based practice experiences. If responsibilities are not defined prior to practice experiences, confusion and chaos may ensue, leading to strained relationships most notably between preceptors, students, facilities, and educational institutions. Responsibilities should be predetermined, hopefully by consensus, defined in writing, and leave little room for misunderstanding. In many cases, the duties of students and preceptors are spelled out via evaluation forms, course syllabi, and other materials made available by the university, the preceptor, and the facility. Various areas addressed within these documents may include, but are not limited to, maintenance of official documents such as time sheets and evaluations; observance of due dates for assignments or other paperwork; preceptor preparation for student arrival; student registration for internship courses; student notification of illness; and many others.

It is the responsibility of the college or school to provide a pharmacy program that meets or exceeds accreditation standards, and is of such quality that graduates of that program may pass licensure exams and become successful practitioners and agents of change for the profession. The responsibilities of the facility and the university and/or college are primarily articulated via educational affiliation agreements, oftentimes developed by entities or departments (legal services, educational resources, human resources) outside of the groups involved. For more information on written agreements, see Chapter 11, "Partnerships with Schools." Periodic meetings between colleges or schools, students, preceptors, and facilities can serve as a forum to review each party's responsibilities. Licensing agencies protect the public through regulation of the profession, and therefore influence how experiential programs operate within the practice community through regulation of preceptors and student interns.

Describing Expectations

Failure to set reasonable and mutually agreeable expectations can result in a disappointing and unfulfilling practice experience for all involved. Students may feel that their rotation or other experience was not educationally rewarding. Preceptors may feel disappointed if their expectations for student performance are not fully realized. The college or school of pharmacy may feel the strain of unmet expectations either from the preceptor, the students, or both. Over time, this can adversely affect relationships critical to the internship experience.

General expectations, like responsibilities, should be described in some detail through evaluation forms, course syllabi, and other materials. For students, these should be defined for professional behavior as well as academic performance by both the educational institution and the preceptor. Core knowledge, skills, attitudes, and values should be defined, articulated, and assessed. A school-based orientation immediately prior to practice experience courses, during which course materials are reviewed and students are prepped for the experience, can help accomplish this goal. Preceptors need to know what the college or school of pharmacy expects from them in the areas of student activities, communication, evaluation, and other aspects of the relationship. This can be achieved within the framework of site visits, periodic group meetings between preceptors and schools, focus groups, etc.

Expectations specific to each practice experience can be individualized between the preceptor and the student. Ideally, this would occur immediately prior to the beginning of each introductory pharmacy practice experience (IPPE) or advanced pharmacy practice experience (APPE) in a meeting between the preceptor and student so that both parties are able to make the best use of the time allotted for the experience. The preceptor's expectations of the student can relate to the following areas: daily schedule and when the student can expect to meet with the preceptor throughout the week; specific responsibilities within the institution and how that translates into opportunities for the students; how the students should interact with other pharmacy and institutional personnel; educational and behavioral goals related to the preceptor's practice; and any specific training or orientation required by the facility prior to the beginning of the rotation. Students should be able to articulate their expectations in the context of their previous experience, desire for exposure in specific areas of the practice, and career goals.

Designing a practice experience, specifically an APPE, that meets the students' professional or career expectations can result in a professionally rewarding experience for both preceptor and students. For example, if a student begins a nutrition rotation and articulates an interest in pursuing this specialized area of pharmacy practice, the preceptor and student are well served by exposing the student maximally to appropriate activities and people who can help this student achieve his or her career goal. Another example is the student who begins an institutional rotation with years of experience in making IVs. This student may assist the preceptor with a special project rather than spending hours in IV training, creating a win-win situation for both parties.

As shown above, the preceptor-student relationship is one that can involve a multitude of individuals and groups. Following the steps described above can set all of these parties on the path to a healthy, long-term, and professionally rewarding relationship.

Motivating and Challenging Students to Enhance Their Performance

Motivational Theory

What motivates students to act, think, and behave in certain ways? What makes students more likely to work hard, achieve, be creative, and complete assignments? Several early motivation theorists have been studied, and their original theories are still the underpinnings of much of today's modern discussions on this topic.

This first group of theorists assumes that all people have needs, expectations, and desires, and that their needs, expectations, and desires must be met if you are to achieve success for your organization (or student rotation in this case). Two of the most popular theories include Maslow's hierarchy of needs theory and Herzberg's two-factor theory.[11] Each needs theory differs somewhat in the needs identified and the explanation of how unfulfilled needs influence motivation. Maslow, for example, states that individuals have five levels of needs arranged in a hierarchical format. The most basic needs include physiological needs and safety needs. The next level is belongingness and love, and the higher needs levels include esteem and self-actualization. Herzberg's theory complements

Maslow's and describes two types of needs factors. The first type is the motivator factor, which satisfies higher-order needs (autonomy, self actualization, self-esteem) and motivates a person to achieve. The second type is the hygiene factor, which satisfies lower-order needs (security, social, salary, benefits) and prevents dissatisfaction.

The second group of theorists bases their work on an equity principle. This principle evolved from social comparison theory. Here, people assess their performance and attitudes by comparing both their contribution to work and the benefits they derive from it to the contributions and benefits of a comparison other. This comparison other may be like or unlike the person (i.e., another classmate with respect to what they are doing in their rotations to achieve success). Reinforcement represents the third grouping of theorists and was prompted by the famous Skinner research. It emphasizes the importance of feedback and rewards in motivating behavior through diverse reinforcement techniques.

Finally, the fourth group of theorists promotes expectancy theory, which is more comprehensive in its approach and integrates many of the elements of needs, equity, and reinforcement theory. Vroom popularized expectancy theory with his model stating that motivation is a function of expectancy, valence, and instrumentality. Expectancy refers to a person's perception of the probability that effort will lead to performance. For example, a person who believes that if he or she works harder then he or she will produce more has a high expectation that hard work leads to productivity. Valence refers to a person's perception of the value of the projected outcomes (that is, how much the person likes or dislikes receiving those outcomes). Instrumentality refers to a person's perception of the probability that certain outcomes (positive or negative) will be attached to performance. For example, the person that sees a link between productivity and greater benefits has high instrumentality.

Application to Student Rotations

Our goal in student rotations is to motivate and challenge students to bring out their best performance. This requires leadership on the part of the preceptor. All students are not at the same point in their development and all students are not at the same motivational level. We want to bring out the best in students by focusing on their behavior and creating consistently high performances. We have to acknowledge that all students will not be outstanding performers, but most students can attain a higher level of achievement. We can use our leadership skills to tap their full potential and get them to perform at higher levels. We create an environment for the student rotation that gives students an advantage to find the road to success. I will suggest three environmental factors that are under your control that will help you to motivate and challenge your students as well as to enhance their performance. As I discuss these three factors, I will also relate them to the previous theories discussed above.

Develop Positive Expectations with Your Students from the Start

Vroom posited his expectancy theory with the factors of instrumentality, valence, and expectations. You need to take a leadership role from the beginning in helping your students think that they can accomplish their rotation goals. This may not be easy. They interact with many other people, and some of their other contacts may have less enthusiasm and lower expectations. Positive expectations are not effective in a vacuum. Students have to be communicated to, understood by, and accepted by everyone on the clinical team that will interact with them.

Expecting much without having positive expectations of the students is a set-up for failure for both parties involved. We all know the power of positive expectations. Now think of the converse situation. If you have shared negative expectations with your students, they have a head start on failure. And remember the methods of communication that are available to send messages: body language, eye contact, and other nonverbal cues. Make sure that your messages of positive expectation to the students are consistent and match your intentions. Your positive expectations must begin from reality. That is, you must assess the baseline of the students prior to defining expectations for the rotation. This again requires effort and leadership on your part. Once you understand the baseline and accept the reality, your positive expectations can have a significant impact on the performance of your students.

Ensure That Students Take Responsibility for Achieving Their Rotation Goals

You are familiar with the old refrain, that if everyone has responsibility for a goal, then no one has responsibility for the goal. Temptation may be to sit around and wait for someone else to take the lead unless assignments and roles are clearly delineated. Make responsibility a positive endeavor. Do not assign as if it is a punishment but rather as an opportunity and challenge to do something good and to show value and worth. Of course, you need clear goals for students. Do not assume that everyone understands the goals. Setting goals with students creates a proactive environment, which helps students to focus on the endpoint of the work. Without that goal and endpoint, students can get caught up in all of the activity without remembering why they started in the first place. The goal setting session is crucial to students.

Every student is different and you need to use a different style for each student. Your mutually defined goals should match each student's course objectives and abilities. If you set the goals too high, students may become demoralized and fail or give up. If you set the goals too low, students may become disinterested and unmotivated. You can decide at what level you want to set the goals, but be aware that the higher the goals are set, the more you should plan to support the students in reaching those goals. Do not march students out to reach stretch or maybe even bigger stretch goals without planning to be there for support. You need to think about that during the goal setting stage, and it is probably obvious to you that students will develop faster with your support. There is some validity to the notion that goals should be set somewhere between too high, where students will have little likelihood of success, and too low, where success is a sure thing. The best goals may be in the area of a high probability of success with challenge still involved.

Ensure that students understand their goals, and ask them to define how you and they will measure success. What is due, when it is due, and what it will look like are all issues that should be in agreement as the rotation begins. Students rarely set out to disappoint their preceptors and mentors—it is often a case of misunderstanding. Another key piece of responsibility is defining the action steps to success. You do this yourself when you take on big projects. Goals are not reached by pure luck, so also ask your students to do this. Help them define their need to visit the library, gain access to the Internet, spend time in a student study group, or participate in daily medical rounds to learn more about their assigned patients. Action steps spell out the big and little steps necessary in reaching rotation-defined goals. A good action-steps document helps ensure success in reaching goals.

Finally, one indirect benefit of all of this activity (assigning responsibility, setting goals, writing action steps), is that it forces students to be interactive, involved, and committed to the rotation. The more involved that students are with planning (with defining responsibilities and identifying goals and action steps), the greater the commitment. Students will know if they are on the right track or if they have fallen off the path and there is need for a correction or adjustment. And the more involved they are, the more responsible they are for the outcomes.

Use Feedback to Motivate Your Students

Be sure to incorporate lots of feedback into student rotations. This will help stimulate, challenge, and motivate your students. Remember that Maslow talks about belongingness, esteem, and self-actualization needs. Herzberg talks about motivators. Too often students demonstrate appropriate behavior and receive either positive feedback, negative feedback, or no feedback at all. Recall again that every student is an individual and different styles of feedback work with different students, and different styles of feedback meet different needs in working with students. Skinner's theory emphasized the importance of feedback and rewards in motivating behavior through diverse reinforcement techniques.

Let's discuss positive feedback first. This involves pairing a desired behavior or outcome with positive reinforcement and feedback. Responding with positive feedback encourages students. It is reinforcing and it motivates students for additional achievement.

Negative feedback brings results that are less predictable. With negative feedback, you are acting to stop a behavior or outcome that has already occurred. The result may encourage students to perform better, but it does not always work that way. Students may feel that they are being punished and may quit trying.

• Preceptor Pearls •

Remember that optimal feedback for good performance should be positive in tone and timely. Withholding feedback can produce mixed results.

Withholding feedback also causes the discontinuation of certain behaviors. Failure to provide positive feedback causes a behavior to cease. Removing positive feedback may contribute to a decline in performance. Withholding feedback may be even more punishing than negative feedback, because it is the least motivating response you can make to any student behavior or performance. And if you ignore a bad performance as if it did not happen, the poor performance is likely to be repeated. Things may even get worse. If you ignore a good performance or even a slightly improved performance, you are going to remove the motivation to improve. Students make additional efforts to improve, and they are not recognized.

Probably the most common type of feedback provided by preceptors is that of withholding feedback, and that is what students dislike the most. Everyone wants attention. Most of us do not recognize how difficult withholding reinforcement can be on students. Sometimes receiving negative reinforcement may even be preferred and may drive students to be recognized in that manner.

Generational Issues to Keep in Mind

While remembering the importance of addressing each student as a unique individual, there are generational issues to keep in mind while working with our current students. While we preceptors may be hailing from the "baby boomer" or "genX" generations, our current generation of students has been referred to as "millenials."[12] Millenials as a group are hard-working, competitive, productive, and have been successful at much of what they have accomplished. They expect to be treated with respect and are open-minded with respect to different races, religions, sexual orientations, and other issues in the workplace. Gender equality was addressed years ago and is no longer an issue. They consider themselves to be global in perspective and are motivated to improve the human condition—in our country and abroad. While they like challenges and stimulation and are capable of multitasking and high technology utilization, they strongly focus on maintaining a work life balance to keep friends and family near and involved. One final note on millenials is that they do like praise. This generation has been praised heavily by parents and teachers alike, and they need and expect this recognition. Consequently, incorporate it into your preceptor style.

A Final Note on Extrinsic Factors and Rewards

Much of this chapter has focused on the intrinsic factors in motivating students. Preceptors are encouraged to develop positive student expectations, invite students to take responsibility for their success, and provide important feedback to students. Do not forget to consider extrinsic factors and utilize extrinsic rewards when appropriate and available. There are simple, inexpensive, and very effective opportunities to help reward and further motivate students. An example might be to invite your students to attend a professional association meeting as your guests. Showing your interest and sharing your time impresses students who look at you as a role model. Also, a simple gift such as a reference text, healthcare-related book, or a stethoscope or other practical tool provides a strong gesture to students.

Summary

Motivational theory can help in a preceptor-student relationship. We need to utilize all available tools to ensure a successful rotation and outcome. Remember that detecting generational differences may provide insights. Even more importantly is to remember that each student is unique and should be addressed as an individual and as the focus of a student centric experience.

Creating an Environment That Promotes a Win-Win-Win Situation for Preceptors, Pharmacist Interns, and Clinical Practice Sites

This section includes information that can be applied to an advanced student experiential opportunity. While this section will help all preceptors in their work with students, it also contains ideas and tools to craft an integrative patient care environment, a well-structured learning environment, and a potential research environment for those preceptors seeking to offer this advanced level of rotation.

An effective and successful clerkship rotation is an arrangement from which the preceptor, pharmacist intern, and clinical practice site derive the greatest benefit. With careful forethought and preplanned orientation activities, the preceptor can create a working environment for the intern that is friendly and fully integrated into the activities of the clinical site. The following pages describe aspects that can help create a working environment that promotes a win-win-win situation for preceptors, pharmacist interns, and clinical practice sites.

Creating an Organized Environment in a Complex Practice

Good rapport with healthcare colleagues and other coworkers is the foundation needed to build a successful preceptorship at the clinical site. Once the preceptor has established credibility in the practice setting and demonstrates value in service, arranging a clerkship rotation for a pharmacist intern can be more readily supported by administrators and endorsed by clinical colleagues and pharmacy/office personnel. Once preceptorship has been approved at the practice site, contact the school of pharmacy to start planning for student rotation opportunities. For example, setting up a clinical rotation for a pharmacist intern in a hospital, community or an ambulatory care environment requires that the preceptor receive an agreement from administrators of the pharmacy (or clinic, hospital, academic department) that grants him or her the time and space needed to precept. Often, the pharmacy (or clinic, hospital, academic department) makes in-kind contributions so that the preceptor can assume teaching responsibilities in addition to his or her routine duties. When directors and managers support the function of teaching activities, the preceptors will likely feel less burdened.[13] Sometimes the workflow of other colleagues is affected. If the clerkship rotation requires that the intern work with a multidisciplinary medical team, the preceptor also needs to inform the attending physician and make proper arrangements with other team members.

Only after the preceptor has fully integrated his or her services into a clinical practice can he or she clearly understand the needs of the practice site. If the preceptor is not clear about his or her role, it will be difficult for him or her to organize an effective clerkship rotation for an intern, meet the intern's learning objectives, and provide networking opportunities for the intern. Every effort should be made to clarify the preceptor's role and to identify the practice site's needs before a preceptorship is undertaken so that the intern's activities will not be perceived to be disruptive.

Once you have begun the initial dialogues between the school and site, leaders can arrange for a site visit to assess the learning environment and review learning objectives for students to evaluate the suitability of this program. You will want to focus on such issues as preceptor availability, evidence of ongoing scholarly activities within the department and hospital, logistics (working space, availability of computers, etc.), and the overall support from the department of pharmacy and hospital for this action. Make sure you bring as many documents as necessary to explain your school's advanced practice experiential education curriculum. You will need to begin discussions concerning a site affiliation agreement between your school and the facility. This can often involve a lengthy process frequently lasting between 6 months and a year. Additionally, be prepared to discuss the intern's preclinical program at your school. This is important because it will give the director some idea of your intern's educational background and level of preparation before starting experiential programs at the facility.

You can also embark on a discussion of the benefits being affiliated with the school of pharmacy. This would include faculty status for preceptors, access to the school library system, preceptor development conferences, and continuing education activities just to name a few. Since it is the first experience for this department of pharmacy and your school, you may initially take a go-slow approach. You may agree on having only a few students participating during that first year. This approach is optimal because it gives you time to evaluate the overall impact of pharmacist interns in their program and the quality of the educational activities occurring in the facility. The last thing you want to do is to overwhelm a young site. You may also mention that several other community hospitals in the area have pharmacist interns who take part in advanced practice educational experiences.

Providing orientation activities for clerkship interns is important, not only because it would help the interns overcome anxiety, but also because it would give interns a practical overview of the rotation and the requirements for its completion. If possible, a flyer or an e-mail announcement should be distributed to introduce interns to everyone at the site prior to the start of their rotations. Including digital photos of the pharmacist interns on the announcements would help staff and other colleagues at the rotation site know whom to greet and welcome. At the start of the rotation, the preceptor should provide clear instructions to interns so they can fulfill administrative requirements, such as obtaining an identification badge, receiving a computer username and password, completing Health Insurance Portability and Accountability Act (HIPAA) training modules, and, if needed for research or quality improvement projects, both HIPAA and human subjects training certifications. An effective orientation includes the following:

- A checklist that includes orientation items and administrative requirements (samples are included in Scenario 2 and Appendix A)
- A syllabus that outlines rotation goals, objectives, topics to be covered during the rotation (e.g., selection of medications for disease-specific management), assignments, and evaluation criteria (a sample is included in Appendix B)
- A policy that covers etiquette and dress codes in the clinical practice (a sample is included in Appendix B)
- A calendar that contains activities and dates of conferences, seminars, and presentations
- A sample of medication review and monitoring forms (a sample is included in Appendix C), SOAP notes, medical records
- Training for appropriate use of health informatics tools such as electronic medical record or computerized provider order entry systems
- Preferred method for answering phone calls or responding to requests from physicians, nurses, patients
- An initial assessment with the preceptor in which the intern self-evaluates his or her skills and states the goals of the rotation (this assessment allows the preceptor and the intern to work together to develop achievable objectives)
- A tour of the office, pharmacy, hospital ward, and/or the clinic
- A period where the intern follows the preceptor during the first few days (have a gradual training plan)

Other colleagues or office staff can help the preceptor accomplish some of the orientation tasks.

For example, the office staff could help the intern obtain an identification badge or computer sign-on privileges. The nursing staff could help the intern understand clinic flow from the point of check-in to the point of checkout. Helping the intern become familiar with the clinical practice site gives the staff the opportunity to welcome the intern and provides the intern with knowledge that allows him/her to be helpful to the staff during the experiential learning process. In a survey of more than 200 physician residents, the investigators found that learning opportunities should be structured so that learners "are oriented to the site, have their knowledge assessed regularly, are helped to meet individual goals, are given appropriate levels of responsibility, and see an adequate number, mix, and continuity of patients."[14]

• Preceptor Pearls •

Take advantage of opportunities to meet with colleges or schools of pharmacy to better understand roles, responsibilities, and expectations, and give input when requested.

Creating a Comfortable Physical Environment

Having a comfortable physical environment will help both the preceptor and the intern attain better and more efficient work flow. A comfortable physician environment such as having a workspace, computer and Internet access, and computerized patient record system access, has been found to be associated with students' satisfaction in the VA Learners' Perceptions Survey.[15] Although many rotation sites have limited office space and few workstations, the benefit of giving the intern a designated work area (even if it is a shared area) promotes teamwork between the preceptor and the intern, gives the intern a sense of identity, helps the intern understand his or her responsibilities, and makes it easier for the preceptor or other staff members to locate the intern when necessary. Likewise, having a designated desk and a computer obviates logistic inconveniences and streamlines workflow. Having a workspace for the intern in the vicinity of the pharmacy allows the intern to be more efficient in providing services to the pharmacy and in completing pharmacy-related or pharmaceutical care-related duties as the rotation progresses.

Creating an Integrative Patient Care Environment

Once the preceptor matches the needs of the intern with those of the practice site, the preceptor can integrate the intern's activities into the clinical practice. The needs of the clinical practice can be assessed by surveying administrators, office staff, and clinical colleagues for ideas and feedback. For example, the administrators may need interns to help with outcomes projects related to drug utilization or cost-effectiveness analyses. Hospital or clinic administrators may benefit from having interns help provide service in areas such as medication reconciliation. In community pharmacies intern participation in medication therapy management (MTM) programs helps the pharmacies with workload challenges. The nursing or pharmacy staffs might benefit from receiving an information handout on certain drugs or an in-service presentation by the intern. The office staff in a clinic might benefit by having pharmacist interns assist with phone calls relating to medication requests or laboratory reports. Other pharmacists or physicians might need help with medical-literature or drug-information computer searches. Pharmacist interns could help physician-residents select appropriate medication regimens that are evidence-based and within safe dosage limits. The preceptor spends time training the intern; the intern, after effective training, can help reduce workload if the preceptor plans strategically.

Another way of integrating interns into clinical practice is to facilitate encounters with actual patients. Having an adequate number and variety of patients is valued by almost all learners.[16] Treating the intern with respect and allowing the intern to participate in a real-time patient encounter, whether in person or on the phone, can help interns gain professional self-confidence and ultimately reduce the preceptor's workload. The preceptor should coach and encourage the intern during initial encounters. Any patient encounter should, of course, be coordinated with colleagues and the clinical staff. An integrative approach (or the "deep approach") that leads to personal understanding has been found to predict most site and preceptor characteristics valued by 532 medical students and 2,939 residents in one study.[17]

• Preceptor Pearls •

Ensure that you and your clinical practice sites (hospital, community pharmacy, etc.) have set mutual goals regarding student education.

Creating a Teaching and Learning Environment

When creating a teaching environment it is imperative that the preceptor and site be equipped with a number of key resources and activities. Among the most important assets are those that are a part of the ongoing staff education and development programs in the institution. The intern should be able to observe and participate in a number of educational actions including journal club discussions, clinical forums, pharmacy work rounds, pharmacy grand rounds, and patient education seminars. As the intern increases participation in these activities, he or she has the opportunity to observe various presentation styles. Through formal and informal presentation assignments, interns can continue to improve their own presentation skills. The preceptor should also involve the intern in nonpharmacy teaching events. The intern should be able to observe and participate in a number of physician and nursing educational events including medical and nursing grand rounds, nursing shift report, medical work rounds, medical journal club, and attending rounds. As the intern becomes more involved in the day-to-day measures of the experience, the preceptor may take the opportunity to provide mentorship to the intern by initiating discussions regarding professional opportunities postpharmacy school, including residency and fellowship opportunities, careers in hospital or ambulatory care pharmacy, pharmaceutical industry, research, or government service.

The pharmacist intern would benefit from having a good learning environment. Learning environment, together with domain factors of the clinical faculty, working environment, and physical environment, have been found to be significantly associated with overall training satisfaction score rating responded by 6,527 medical students and 16,583 physician residents in the VA Learners' Perceptions Survey.[15] The survey found that the learning environment domain, including items such as preparation for future training and quality of care, had the strongest association with overall training satisfaction score.[15] In addition, a good learning environment is where the preceptor pays attention to pharmacist interns during their career developmental stage. This does not mean, however, that the preceptor needs to spend every minute of their work time with interns. Rather, interns usually enjoy working independently while receiving tips from the preceptor and being incorporated to the healthcare team at the experiential site. We recommend that the preceptor ask interns about their expectations for the rotation and, if possible, tailor the rotation contents to meet the individual intern's professional development needs while maintaining a win-win-win situation for the pharmacist intern, the preceptor, and the clinical practice site.

Creating a Practice-Based Research Environment

Understanding the intern's professional-development needs at the time of the rotation can help the preceptor design a better rotation program for the individual intern. If the intern wants to learn more about case studies, the preceptor can help the intern develop skills in this area and even write up formal clinical case reports. If the intern wants to learn about research and scientific writing, the preceptor can work with the intern to develop research protocols, or prepare poster abstracts and manuscripts for publication. Such a focus requires that the preceptor be knowledgeable about research procedures and have scholarly discipline. If the preceptor or his/her department offers a residency program for pharmacists, and if the intern is interested in pursuing residency training, the rotation in such an integrative environment can be an opportunity for both to see if they have found a good match.

Activities such as discussions in journal club meetings or activities related to research efforts that produce deliverables such as preliminary data or manuscripts would benefit both the preceptors and the pharmacist interns who would like to participate in these efforts. Practice-based research identifies, studies, and evaluates common problems encountered in clinical practice.[18] Collaboratively engaging in practice-based research projects gives the pharmacist intern an opportunity to see how research efforts could improve the quality and safety of care; the pharmacist intern benefits the preceptor and clinical site by helping to collect and analyze data that are used to improve pharmacy operation, clinical outcomes, patient satisfaction, and staff efficiency. Practice-based research questions arise from the practice; study findings could be used by the practice to re-engineer the practice operations, increase appropriate medication use, and explore additional ways to further improve medication safety.[18]

Creating Intern Interest in Preceptorship

The preceptor has a golden opportunity to imbue the intern with the expectation that he or she will want to become a preceptor. The preceptor can do this in several ways. First and foremost, by consistently demonstrating a positive attitude when working with the intern shows the intern that the preceptor derives both personal and professional pleasures from being a preceptor. The preceptor can influence the intern by displaying enthusiasm for teaching and by maintaining excellent scholarship. This shows the intern that clinical effectiveness can be maintained and improved through teaching and precepting. The intern will then recognize that this state of readiness is necessary to ensure consistently positive patient outcomes. The preceptor can influence the interns' expectations for becoming a preceptor by providing the intern with meaningful patient care assignments in which they are expected to be key decision makers. Lastly, the preceptor, by taking an interest in some of the interns' professional interests and incorporating the intern into the practice site in a collegial manner, shows the intern that preceptorship is a collaborative endeavor with the intern being an important part of the partnership.

Creating a Networking Environment That Extends Beyond Rotation

The preceptor can help the pharmacist interns identify opportunities for professional networking by linking them with local or national professional societies. The preceptor can share with the interns his/her involvement in committee work, local pharmacy operations, leadership activities, community service, and/or practice-based research experiences. Witnessing the efforts the preceptor makes towards collaborative research projects that help improve the quality and safety of patient care and pharmacy operations could help the intern gain an appreciation of collaborative research contributions and networking advantages with other pharmacist peers. Through networking efforts, the preceptor and the pharmacist intern work together to forge a longer working bond that could potentially benefit sites beyond the experiential training site.

Summary

A win-win-win situation for preceptors, pharmacist interns, and clinical practice sites can be created from an organized environment that also provides a comfortable, physical workspace. Having an integrative patient care setting, where both teaching and learning activities occur to address training needs and career development for both the preceptor and the pharmacist intern, is beneficial for both. Stretching clinical tasks to include collaborative practice-based research efforts that improve outcomes, efficiencies, and satisfactions for those affected by the experiential site can be a rewarding experience for the pharmacist intern, preceptor, and the clinical practice site. The influence that the preceptor has on the pharmacist intern undoubtedly extends beyond experiential rotations and brings benefits to career developments for both.

Chapter Summary

Many factors contribute to a successful practice experience for the student and to a rewarding professional experience for both the student and preceptor. Understanding the roles and responsibilities of both parties is vital and appreciating each others' perspectives is helpful too. Preceptors can increase the likelihood of a successful practice experience with effective planning and by optimizing the practice environment. Effective utilization of feedback and motivation techniques further enhance the chances of a successful experience.

References

1.   Grasha A, Richlin L. *Teaching with Style*. Pittsburgh, PA: Alliance Publishers; 1996.

2.   Whitman N, Schwenk TL. *Preceptors as Teachers: A Guide to Clinical Teaching*. Salt Lake City, UT: University of Utah School of Medicine; 1984.

3.   American Association of Colleges of Pharmacy Academic-Practice Partnership Initiative. Pilot project to profile exemplary advanced practice experience sites. September 14, 2006. Available at: http://www.aacp.org/resources/education/APPI/Documents/Pilot%20Project%20PPEs.pdf.

4.   Bell HS, Kozakowski SM. Teaching the new competencies using the gap analysis approach. *Fam Med.* 2006 Apr;38(4):238–9.

5.   Koenigsfeld CF, Tice AL. Organizing a community advanced pharmacy practice experience. *Am J Pharm Educ.* 2006 Feb 15;70(1):22.

6.   Collins JC, Porras JI. *Built to Last: Successful Habits of Visionary Companies.* New York, NY: HarperCollins Publishers; 1997.

7.   Ende J. Feedback in clinical medical education. *JAMA.* 1983 Aug 12;250(6):777–81.

8.   Hammer D. Improving student professionalism during experiential learning. *Am J Pharm Educ.* 2006 Jun 15;70(3):59.

9.   American Pharmacists Association. Code of Ethics for Pharmacists. October 27, 1994. Available at: http://www.pharmacist.com/AM/Template.cfm?Section=Search1&template=/CM/HTMLDisplay.cfm&ContentID=2903. Accessed December 29, 2008.

10. Accreditation Council for Pharmacy Education. *Accreditation Standards and Guidelines for the Professional Program in Pharmacy Leading to the Doctor of Pharmacy Degree.* Chicago, IL: Accreditation Council for Pharmacy Education; 2006. Available at: http://www.acpe-accredit.org/pdf/ACPE_Revised_PharmD_Standards_Adopted_Jan 152006.pdf.

11. Gibson JL, Ivancevich JM, Donnelly JH, et al. *Organizations: Behavior, Structure, Processes.* 6th ed. New York, NY: McGraw Hill/Irwin; 1988:109–31.

12. Orrell L. *Millenials Incorporated: The Big Business of Recruiting, Managing and Retaining North America's New Generation of Young Professionals.* 1st ed. Deadwood, OR: Intelligent Women Publishing, Wyatt-MacKenzie; 2007.

13. Kemper NJ. Win-win strategies help relieve preceptor burden. *Nurs Manage.* Feb 2007;38(2):10.

14. Roth LM, Severson RK, Probst JC, et al. Exploring physician and staff perceptions of the learning environment in ambulatory residency clinics. *Fam Med.* Mar 2006;38(3):177–84.

15. Cannon GW, Keitz SA, Holland GJ, et al. Factors determining medical students' and residents' satisfaction during VA-based training: findings from the VA Learners' Perceptions Survey. *Acad Med.* Jun 2008;83(6):611–20.

16. Schultz KW, Kirby J, Delva D, et al. Medical Students' and Residents' preferred site characteristics and preceptor behaviours for learning in the ambulatory setting: a cross-sectional survey. *BMC Med Educ.* Aug 6 2004;4:12.

17. Delva MD, Schultz KW, Kirby JR, et al. Ambulatory teaching: do approaches to learning predict the site and preceptor characteristics valued by clerks and residents in the ambulatory setting? *BMC Med Educ.* 2005;5:35.

18. Kuo GM, Steinbauer JR, Spann SJ. Conducting medication safety research projects in a primary care physician practice-based research network. *J Am Pharm Assoc (2003).* 2008;48(2):163–70.

Appendix A. Orientation Checklist for the Pharmacist Intern (sample)

Rotation (type and name): xxx
Site: xxx Pharmacy
Preceptor: Name and Contact Information

1. First Day of Rotation

- ❑ Meet at preceptor's office for the orientation packet.
- ❑ Take a tour of the facility.
- ❑ Obtain an ID/security card.
- ❑ Obtain computer access ID and password.
- ❑ Try computer access. Consult the department's IT office for computer related questions (list IT contact person and phone number).
- ❑ Fill out EMR (electronic medical record) application forms to get ID and password.
- ❑ Take the online HIPAA and security training courses (list website address and contact person's name, phone number, and e-mail if there are questions). Complete the courses and exams, and print out the certificate on completion.
- ❑ Take the online Human Research Certification Exams (list website address and contact person's name, phone number, and e-mail if there are questions). Complete the modules and exams, and print out the certificates on completion.
- ❑ Review the following disease states and pharmacotherapy (for primary care rotation): diabetes; hypertension; hypercholesterolemia; and anticoagulation.
- ❑ Review information on MTMS reimbursement billing codes. Reference: http://www.pharmacist.com/AM/Template.cfm?Section=Newsroom&TEMPLATE=/CM/HTMLDisplay.cfm&CONTENTID=14126. Review information on reimbursement for collaborative cognitive service (pharmaceutical care). Reference: Kuo GM, Buckley TE, Fitzsimmons D, et al. Collaborative drug therapy management services and reimbursement in a family medicine clinic (special feature article). *Am J Health Syst Pharm.* 2004;61:343–54.
- ❑ Familiarize with primary care quality improvement projects (varies with institutional focus and emphasis each year):
  - Evidence-based clinical guideline adherence
  - Chronic disease management
  - Medication safety

2. First Week of Rotation

- ❑ Complete all training modules and certification exams.

- ❑ Learn to use the following programs:
  - EMR—practice reviewing patient charts
  - Medical library links (including PubMed searches and drug information resources)
  - Reference software (e.g., Endnote) program
  - Microsoft Word, Excel, Access, and Powerpoint
- ❑ Start selecting articles to review and present at journal clubs during the rotation.
- ❑ Start writing SOAP notes and/or pharmacotherapy consultation notes.
- ❑ Select a research or quality improvement project.
- ❑ Turn in initial self-assessment (evaluation form).

3. Throughout the Rotation

- ❑ Fulfill rotation requirements as outlined in the rotation handbook.
- ❑ Complete mid-rotation self-assessment and evaluation
- ❑ Complete daily or weekly assignments (patient case, journal critique)
- ❑ Ask questions.
- ❑ Continue working on a clinical improvement and/or a research project.

4. End of Rotation

- ❑ Fulfill rotation requirements as outlined in the rotation handbook.
- ❑ Turn in all assignments (patient case, journal critique, final project/paper).
- ❑ Complete end-of-rotation self-assessment and evaluation.

Appendix B. Rotation Syllabus for the Pharmacist Intern (sample)

Elective Rotation in Family Medicine

The 6-week rotation provides an opportunity for pharmacist intern to experience family medicine as practiced in urban areas in xxx. Each student will be supervised by the preceptor, xxx, who is practicing in the xxx clinic serving (the rotation site).

Rotation Description

Family Medicine (M–F, 7:30 a.m.–4 p.m.)

Supervised advanced professional education in a family medicine clinic emphasizing pharmaceutical care and evidence-based pharmacotherapy. Interns will assess, evaluate, and monitor therapy of acute and chronic diseases encountered in family medicine and provide drug information to patients and other healthcare practitioners.

Rotation Goals and Objectives

Goal: The intern will develop an understanding of the unique nature of primary care in family medicine clinics, serving urban patients including underserved population; the intern will gain experience and develop competence in providing clinical and operational functions in primary care.

Objectives: The intern will

1. Assume personal responsibility for attaining excellence in one's own ability to provide primary care.
2. Display initiative in preventing, identifying, and resolving therapeutic problems in the primary care setting.
3. Identify and demonstrate basic knowledge of most common patient problems seen in the practice.
4. Identify and demonstrate understanding of pharmacotherapies of commonly encountered diseases/conditions in the practice: (e.g., diabetes, hypertension, hyperlipidemia).

Goal: The intern will establish professional relationships with patients as well as other healthcare professionals and staffs at the clinic.

Objectives: The intern will

1. Provide drug information effectively through both verbal and written communication to patients at the clinic as well as follow-up phone calls or e-mails.
2. Provide drug information effectively through both verbal and written communication to other healthcare professionals via chart documentation and presentations.

Goal: The intern will participate in the examination, evaluation and management of patients in the practice, and will evaluate several clinical problems in depth.

Objectives: The intern will

1. Collect and evaluate patient data to determine appropriate pharmaceutical care for clinic patients:

   - Generate chronologically-based medication history, including natural/herbal/dietary supplements.

   - Perform vital signs exams as well as appropriate physical examinations to monitor patients' medication use.

   - Interpret laboratory test results in order to assess patient compliance and monitor medication regimens.

   - Evaluate information from the patient's electronic medical records to make decisions on meeting a patient's healthcare needs.

   - Organize patient data into a format that facilitates making clinical decisions.

2. Design, implement, monitor, evaluate, and modify patient pharmacotherapy with evidence-based medicine approach to ensure effective, safe, and economical patient care:

   - Integrate patient disease and drug data to determine desired therapeutic outcomes for a patient by using effective interviewing skills and performing appropriate physical assessment.

   - Discuss and consider patients' risk factors when determining therapeutic outcomes.

   - Formulate an optimal pharmacotherapeutic regimen by selecting patient-specific drug, dose, dosage form, route of administration, schedule, and duration of therapy.

   - Design and implement a method for a pharmacotherapeutic plan based on the purpose of the medication(s), concurrent disease(s) and drug therapies; pharmacokinetic parameters of the drug(s); cost effectiveness; formulary or protocol restrictions; and the patient's clinical condition.

   - Assume responsibility for monitoring patients and judge the continued effectiveness of their therapeutic plan in achieving optimal therapeutic outcomes.

   - Determine the extent to which patients adhere to therapeutic plans.

   - Detect adverse drug reactions and drug-drug, drug-laboratory test, drug-diet, drug-disease and drug-condition interactions and assess their impact on desired therapeutic outcomes.

   - Develop and recommend appropriate revisions to therapeutic plans when optimal therapeutic outcomes are not achieved

   - Document recommendations and patient care activities.

   - Use effective strategies to influence the healthcare behavior of patients toward preventative care.

Goal: The intern will refine self-directed and lifelong learning skills, particularly the ability to access and use biomedical information systems.

Objectives: The intern will

1. Develop and use self-directed learning skills, using resources of the clinical practice site, the medical Library, and the Internet, to better understand the provision of healthcare to patients and to provide evidence-based pharmacotherapy information to other healthcare professionals.

2. Retrieve, analyze, and interpret the professional, lay, and scientific literature to provide drug information to patients, caregivers, health professionals, and the public.

3. Provide concise, applicable, and timely responses for drug information from healthcare providers and patients.

4. Examine clinical and research literature for appropriateness, accuracy, and completeness; evaluate drug studies in the literature in terms of research methodology, validity of results, and clinical applicability through critiques of current pharmacotherapy information during journal club discussions.

Goal: During the rotation the intern will become familiar with clinic operations and consultative services.

Objectives: The intern will

1. Demonstrate understanding of how a family medicine clinic is operated (e.g., scheduling clinic appointments, patient waiting time, medical record retrieval, clinic assessment and examinations, prescribing medications, system for refilling medications, chart documentation, charging fee-for-service).

2. Learn and practice patient care in both inpatient services and clinics and to appreciate continuity in patient care.

3. Demonstrate understanding of when and why consultations are sought, how consultants and consultative services are chosen.

4. Appreciate the clinical importance of interdisciplinary care for clinic patients.

5. Demonstrate understanding of appropriate communication among providers, consultants and patients.

Goal: The intern will participate in scholarly activities through research or quality improvement projects and clinical write-ups.

Objectives: The intern will

1. Design, conduct, and complete a research/QI project relevant to the practice in family medicine OR

2. Complete an evidence-based pharmacotherapy write-up or a case report ready for publication.

Rotation Activities and Assignments

The intern is expected to participate in all practice settings as assigned; conduct clinical practice with professional mannerism; monitor and manage patients' medication regimens; document and review all interventions with the preceptor; present all patient cases verbally and in pharmaceutical consult notes or SOAP note format; show understanding of diseases/conditions encountered in the clinic; attend conferences and discussions; discuss and participate in journal clubs; design and conduct research projects in family medicine or complete a formal clinical write-up; and perform self-evaluations at the beginning, middle, and the end of rotations.

A. Clinical Practice

- Interviewing patients for medication histories
- Monitoring medication regimens and developing drug therapy plans to achieve optimal therapeutic outcomes
- Counseling patients on medications and chronic disease management
- Assessing drug-drug, drug-food, drug-lab test interactions
- Interpreting laboratory test results
- Identifying and discerning the nature, severity, and clinical significance of adverse drug reactions
- Documenting all clinical interventions and assessing outcomes of these interventions
- Presenting patient cases and therapeutic recommendations to faculty physicians, medical interns, and nursing staff

B. Scholarly Activities

- Completing a research/QI project or a formal clinical write-up
- Weekly disease summary write-ups
- Patient case presentations daily and in consultation or SOAP notes
- Completing drug information requests as needed
- Two to three journal club presentations during the rotation

C. Conferences and meetings (please check with preceptor for dates)

Dress Code and Professional Manner

A professional appearance must be maintained at all times. Interns are expected to come to work appropriately attired and maintain a professional appearance at all times. All interns must wear a white coat with nameplate and ID cards. Interns are to sign in and out at the beginning and the end of the day. Interns need to notify the preceptor in case of delayed arrival to the clinic.

The clinic is located in a building occupied with many professional people. The manner in which we dress directly impacts how we are perceived by the public, our fellow coworkers, and how we feel about our job responsibilities (adapted from the xxx Family Medicine Clinic Policy).

The following attire is acceptable during regular working hours:

WOMEN

Dresses
Suits with skirts, slacks
Blouses/sweaters with skirts/slacks
Business shoes
Business wear stockings or socks

MEN

Collared buttondown shirts
Dress slacks
Suits, sweaters, sports jackets
Business shoes
Socks (required)

The following attire will **NOT** be acceptable for **men or women** during regular working hours:

Miniskirts (over 2 ½" above the knee)
Jeans
Sneakers or tennis shoes
T-shirts
Spandex, skin tight and/or revealing sheer clothing
Shorts
Caps, hats, or head coverings
Tank or halter tops
Revealing necklines
Note: Skirts and short suits cannot be shorter than 2 ½" above the knee.

Evaluations

The intern must perform self-evaluations at the beginning, the middle and the end of the rotation; evaluations from the preceptor will be conducted during the 3rd (mid-rotation) and 6th week (the final week) of the rotation.

Appendix C. Pharmacotherapy Worksheet (sample)

xxx Rotation

Patient: _____ Age _____ Gender _____

PCP _____ Date: _____

CC: _____ Vitals: Ht _____ Wt _____

BMI _____ B/P _____ P _____ RR _____

PROBLEM	Medication	Dose	Potential SE	Lab (Date)	Monitoring	Therapy Goal

Allergies (medication/reaction):

A/P:

Every great man is always being helped by everybody;
for his gift is to get good out of all things and persons.
John Ruskin

Chapter 4

Mentors

Debra S. Devereaux

Chapter Outline

Learning Objectives

- Compare the characteristics of a preceptor relationship with those of a mentoring relationship.
- Recognize traits that are important in order to be an effective mentor.
- Create an environment conducive to mentoring.
- Introduce the student to professionalism.
- Identify qualities in the student that are important for a successful mentoring relationship.
- Identify the rewards that mentoring offers.
- List behaviors that detract from a mentor-student relationship.
- Identify the personal and professional challenges of being a mentor.

By the time we are adults, most of us can identify people who have had a significant influence on our learning and development in our professional and/or personal life. Many of these people have served as mentors, either formally or informally. For hundreds of years, mentoring has been used as a method for handing down knowledge, maintaining culture, supporting talent, and securing future leadership.[1] Research indicates the mentoring process is linked to career success, personal growth, and increased organizational productivity. Mentoring is a journey that enables the student to develop both professionally and personally. This chapter will describe the many roles that mentors play in guiding growth and development and highlight the qualities that are important in both the mentor and the student or mentee.

Comparison of the Preceptor Relationship and the Mentoring Relationship

Have you ever noticed that at the beginning of any book you read (including textbooks) there's an acknowledgement section where the author thanks individuals who have enabled and supported them during the time they wrote the book? It is a rare person who is not indebted to many others for their accomplishments and achievements. Some people have provided support and encouragement on a personal level—family, friends, and significant others. Others have provided professional expertise by listening to ideas, reviewing concepts, sharing expertise, and providing constructive criticism. The latter were probably either in a preceptor role or served as a mentor.

There are many similarities between a precepting relationship and a mentoring relationship. Formal mentoring programs most closely resemble a preceptor relationship. In any formal mentoring program, a mentee may be assigned a mentor, or the mentee and mentor may choose each other. Formal mentoring models are authoritarian because they are introduced and controlled by a senior manager. This model normally occurs in a work environment in which a senior employee with more experience will help orient a new employee. A formal mentoring relationship also usually has a defined duration. At the end of 6 months or 1 year, for example, the formal reporting requirements and orientation period might end. In this way, a precepted rotation is an example of a formal mentoring program because the student is assigned to a service where there is a pharmacist preceptor in charge. The objectives of a formal mentoring program and a preceptor relationship can even be the same, such as indoctrination to the organization culture, department protocol, and the transferring of knowledge.

Occasionally a precepting relationship may evolve into a mentoring relationship when both the preceptor and the student desire to continue their collaboration. The student may admire and wish to emulate the preceptor's career path, commitment to his/her career, expertise, and position. The preceptor may find that his/her interactions with the student are productive, fulfilling, and stimulate him/her to transfer their knowledge and expertise. The mentoring relationship then becomes voluntary for both the student and the preceptor. That is in essence the difference between a preceptor and a mentoring relationship; preceptors and students are assigned, and mentors and mentees are mutually agreed upon.

• Preceptor Pearls •

Experiment with process. Use coaching, role playing, simulations, brainstorming, or try a change of scenery by going for a walk together or attending a sporting event.

Important Qualities in an Effective Mentor

In almost any memoir or autobiography you read, the subject refers to several individuals who provided significant and timely support or who had a major influence in the subject's life either by the example they set or the teaching they provided. In some cases, these relationships were happenstance and occurred through dumb luck or serendipity. In other cases, the subject sought out these individuals because they recognized a need that the other person could fill. A mentoring Hall of Fame would include Yoda and Luke Skywalker in *Star Wars,* Dumbledore and Harry Potter from the *Harry Potter* series, Earl and Tiger Woods, Dick Cheney and George W. Bush, Warren Buffett and Bill Gates, and Brooke Astor and Annette de la Renta. Some of these mentoring relationships were obviously more positive and had better outcomes than others. As mentees seek a productive mentoring relationship, certain factors and considerations would include the following[2]:

- Is the mentor going to support personal or professional development? Or both?
- Have other students had positive experiences with the mentor?
- Has the mentor served as an advocate for students?
- Are the mentor's areas of interest consistent with that of the student?
- What has the mentor achieved in his/her career?
- Will the mentor have time to devote to the relationship?

- Does the mentor have a professional network that will facilitate development of future relationships for the student?
- Will the mentor challenge the student and also be able to nurture him or her?
- Will the mentor create an environment where the student feels at ease to discuss concerns and fears?

Mentor as a Coach and an Advisor

Your role as a mentor will take on many forms as the relationship develops. First and foremost is serving as a coach and an advisor by providing direction as the student learns about the profession of pharmacy. The *Merriam-Webster Dictionary* definition of a coach is a private tutor or one who instructs or trains a team of performers. Used as a verb the definition of "to coach" is to instruct, direct, or prompt. Most often we think of a successful coach as one who wins or coaches his team to victory. A coach in the mentoring model is concerned with the success of an individual and the attainment of personal goals or a personal "win." As the mentor, your role is to guide the student through his or her learning experience and potential career pathways rather than to directly tell the student what he or she should do. In order to be effective in this role, you must be present, mentally and physically. Being present mentally means that you take the time to focus on the student and listen without seeming to be preoccupied or distracted with other responsibilities so that the student feels comfortable and is able to open up.[3] Remember to practice the good listening skills described in Chapter 2.

• Preceptor Pearls •

The amount of time spent listening should be at least four times the amount spent talking.

Creating open communication is essential in order to break down barriers that inevitably exist since the preceptor-student relationship is traditionally perceived by the student as a hierarchy. A key strategy is to demonstrate vulnerability by sharing your personal experiences, including challenges you have experienced, mistakes you have made, and the lessons you have learned. As a result of this process, you will build trust with the student, and the student will feel comfortable sharing his or her feelings with you. This enables you to begin the mentoring process and serve as coach and an advisor to the student. Through ongoing open communication, you can help the student discover his or her strengths and weaknesses, talents and skills, and likes and dislikes. Your role is also to encourage the mentee to confront challenges and take risks by communicating your support and confidence in the student.[3] As a mentor, you play an essential role in helping the mentee develop confidence and self-esteem.

Mentor as a Guide

As a mentor, you also serve as a guide to the mentorship by introducing the student to individuals within the field of pharmacy and to other healthcare professionals within your own organization.

This enables the student to see how different aspects of pharmacy come together and understand the key role that pharmacists play in ensuring the safety of the medication use process. As a result, the mentee may meet new potential mentors who can serve as role models both now and in the future.

Your role is also to introduce the student to pharmacy professional organizations and to provide opportunities for getting involved in the profession, networking, and learning about different career options. If you are able to actually attend a professional meeting with the student, you will have the opportunity to show the student how to network with others in the profession. Your role as guide is to enable the student to discover the many possibilities within pharmacy. Through this process, you will support the student's development of a sense of pride in becoming a pharmacist and the motivation to become involved in the profession.[3]

Mentor as the Role Model

The mentor also serves as a role model who, besides possessing a strong knowledge base, demonstrates caring, passion, a sense of humor, and integrity. Caring and compassion are important aspects of every human relationship and even more so in creating a bond between yourself and the student.

It is important to remember that these qualities may appear to be absent during busy times or when external factors are creating a stressful situation for you. Communicating to the student that you are preoccupied with something—without necessarily having to share specifics—is important so that the student recognizes something else is going on. This acknowledgement also shows the student, by example, the importance of communication about factors impacting the quality of one's interactions with others.

The ideal mentor is passionate about pharmacy and also about the many opportunities that pharmacists have to demonstrate value by improving management of chronic diseases, preventing medication errors, and serving as a resource to other healthcare professionals and patients. When asked what an important quality of a mentor is, the student will usually list a sense of humor since it makes them feel more comfortable and contributes to a positive mentor-mentee relationship.[3]

• Preceptor Pearls •

Focus on wisdom. Be a resource, catalyst, facilitator, idea generator, networker, or problem-solver.

As a mentor you need to be willing to share your knowledge and experience without instructing the student on what to do in a given situation. You may provide suggestions and advice using phrases like "If I was in your position," or "Here's something you might consider," or "Whatever you think will work best, you do." You should utilize methods that rely on asking questions and asking for plans. You should encourage your mentee to brainstorm—there are no bad ideas.

• Preceptor Pearls •

A mentor is not a person with the answers.

It is important to discuss values with the student since it is not uncommon for patient care issues to test the student's value. Values are of particular importance in the pharmacy profession because of the key role we play in patient safety. Examples of situations where value issues are involved include an order for a medication where there is insufficient data regarding efficacy and a potential concern about safety; an expensive drug ordered in a patient without insurance coverage; and a mandate to reduce expenses, which would result in staffing reductions and jeopardize patient safety. Having discussions about value conflicts is an important contribution to the student's growth and understanding of how to deal with difficult issues.[3]

Finally, mentors play an important role in introducing students to the importance of—and the satisfaction that comes with—being committed to lifelong learning. They can do this by sharing recent articles from the scientific or healthcare literature with the student and taking time to discuss some of the key points that were addressed. The mentor may want to introduce the student to a professional organization that combines continuing education programming with networking opportunities. The mentor may also encourage the student to submit the results of projects in poster formats to professional meetings.

Student Attributes

In order for the relationship to be successful, there are a number of characteristics necessary in the mentee.[4] The student needs to be mentorable, which means possessing qualities such as intellectual curiosity, initiative, motivation, and follow-through. The student must be ready to be a partner in the relationship by showing interest in communicating with the mentor and asking for guidance. In many ways, the student's commitment to the relationship is very similar to that of the mentor; he or she needs to invest the time, share experiences, and engage in open and honest dialogue. The student also needs to follow through on tasks or recommendations; otherwise, the mentor will feel that the relationship is not reciprocal.[2] However, even more essential is the student's readiness to learn. The student must do his or her part to build a relationship with the mentor by being responsive to communications and giving the mentor feedback regularly. One could argue here that if the right mentor was chosen, the student is ready. This is true; however, sometimes even though the mentor and student are seemingly compatible, the student has too many other priorities or is not yet at a stage of maturity where he or she is ready to be mentored.[3] If this is the case, the timing for a mentoring relationship is not optimal and should either be postponed or initiated at a time when both parties can be committed to it.

• Preceptor Pearls •

Be patient. Don't always rush into the silence. Silence can stimulate the student.

Mentor-Student Relationship

The mentor-student relationship must have some degree of reciprocity, in which both individuals experience growth and self-discovery. In order for the relationship to be successful, both parties must find it beneficial and feel that their time together was valuable. The mentor-student relationship is one that nurtures both the heart and the mind.[5] The quality of the interaction is based on mutual respect, openness, and honesty. The mentor guides students by weaving together his or her own strengths, weaknesses, likes, and dislikes with those of the students, and in doing so, helps students discover themselves. The mentor serves as advisor, counselor, coach, therapist, guide, and companion.[3] Both the mentor and the student should be changed by the experience. The mentor may have helped the student to uncover an unrecognized or dormant attribute, ability, or talent. The student may be inspired to shift the direction of his or her professional life in a constructive way. The student may have caused the mentor to question long held beliefs and gain new understanding or a new outlook on his or her career. The mentor may feel a sense of renewal and rejuvenation in being a pharmacist. The mentor may feel both personal and professional satisfaction for making a significant contribution to the profession and/or organization.

Studies have shown that students in successful mentoring relationships have a positive attitude toward their work and perceive less stress than individuals without a mentor. A dynamic mentoring relationship allows the student to grow and eventually become an equal of his/her mentor and go on to be a mentor to others.

Challenges of Mentoring

It is important to remember that time constraints will be the most significant barrier to a successful mentoring relationship. Mentors and students have work and life responsibilities that make adding new activities difficult. Especially at the beginning of a mentoring relationship there needs to be a commitment of time and energy to the relationship. Individual thinking and private examination further along in the mentoring relationship will need less time spent together.

Students need feedback, evaluation, and challenges. A mentor needs to strike a balance between support and stretching beyond the student's abilities. The mentor should try not to point out the right and wrong of what a mentee does but rather understand the thought process that led to the decision. The mentor is interested in the reasoning behind the mentee's thinking rather than trying to fix it for him or her.

The student should challenge the mentor's thinking. He or she should make the mentor think about why they decided to become a pharmacist; what it was like starting out; and how they dealt with challenges in their work or personal life.

The mentor and the student should use common sense in avoiding boundary violations such as gift giving, finding the student a new job or promotion, loaning money, or fraternizing. A trusting, caring relationship where both parties maintain privacy, honesty, and integrity is key in a mentoring relationship. Conversations in the relationship are confidential.

A mentoring relationship IS

- A voluntary commitment of both the student and the mentor
- A coaching relationship grounded in sincerity and integrity

- A responsibility
- A learning and growth experience for both parties

A mentoring relationship is NOT

- A social relationship
- A remedial relationship
- A tutoring arrangement
- A recruitment tool

A mentoring relationship can last 2 to 5 years or a lifetime. There are natural ebbs and flows in which one or the other person is more invested in the relationship, and there are different mentoring needs as a person progresses through his or her professional life.

In the most rewarding mentoring relationships, the mentor and the student have mutually identified each other. The mentor may see the student as a younger version of himself or herself. The student may see the mentor as a role model. However, the key to a successful match is not how similar the mentor and the student are but how committed they both are to the relationship. Ideally, the mentor will be able to provide just the right help to the student at just the right time. The mentor is holding up the mirror for the mentee's future pharmacy career. The mentor will help the student to craft a vision for their future pharmacy professional life and assist the mentee in seeing their place in the "big pharmacy picture." And finally, a successful mentoring relationship will have both parties acknowledging the contribution of the other in their as yet unwritten autobiography.

• Preceptor Pearls •

A mentor's role is to "hold up the mirror" for students. A mentor asks questions rather than giving answers.

References

1. Darwin A. Critical reflections on mentoring in work settings. *Adult Education Quarterly.* 2002;50(3):197–211.

2. Hoffman B. Mentoring: on having one and being one. ACCP. Available at: http://www.aacp.org/site/tertiary.asp?TRACKID=&VID=2&CID=513&DID=3939. Accessed January 29, 2004.

3. Shane RR. Finding the right blends in a mentor-student relationship. In: Cuellar LM, Ginsburg DB, eds. *Preceptor's Handbook for Pharmacists.* Bethesda, MD: American Society for Health-System Pharmacists; 2005.

4. APEGGA. Mentoring: attributes of a receptive protégé. Available at: http://www.apegga.org/publications/guidelines/mentor/student.htm. Accessed January 29, 2004.

5. Wilthire SF. Athena's disguises. In: *Mentors in Everyday Life.* Louisville, KY: Westminster John Knox Press; 1999.

Tell me and I will forget. Show me and I may remember. Involve me and I will understand.

Chinese Proverb

Chapter 5

Goals of Experiential Teaching

Dale E. English II, Linda Stevens Albrecht, Ruth E. Nemire, Traci L. Metting

Chapter Outline

Learning Objectives

- Define experiential education and the Accreditation Council for Pharmacy Education standards.

- Utilize the principles of experiential education and engagement of students in "real-life" activities and consequences.

- Discern nuances of cognitive, behavioral, and affective learning.

- Employ the basics of Bloom's taxonomy when developing objectives and assignments.

- Implement a student-centered approach to learning.

- Define lifelong learning.

- Instill the importance of competence through lifelong learning habits.

- Provide appropriate leadership through example.

- Provide basic understanding and utility of continuous professional development (CPD).

- Describe the importance of workplace skills.

- List the five workplace skill competencies.

- Provide examples of how to provide opportunities to understand each of the workplace skill competencies to the students.

Definition of Experiential Teaching

The Association of Experiential Education defines experiential education as "a philosophy and methodology in which educators purposefully engage with learners in direct experience and focused reflection in order to increase knowledge, develop skills and clarify values."[1] Standard No. 14 of the Accreditation Standards and Guidelines for the Professional Program in Pharmacy Leading to the Doctor of Pharmacy Degree requires that pharmacy schools provide practice experiences throughout the curriculum. These pharmacy practice experiences must "integrate, apply, reinforce, and advance the knowledge, skills, attitudes, and values developed through the other components of the curriculum."[2] This standard embodies the definition of experiential education and requires that a significant portion of pharmacy student education be provided through direct experience in practice settings. As preceptors, we assume a vital and necessary role in this process. We are the experiential educators that provide and oversee students in real-life pharmacy settings.

The Association of Experiential Education offers 12 principles of experiential education practice (Box 5.1). A review of these principles compels both teacher and student to take on quite different roles from those assumed in the traditional classroom setting. It also changes how teachers and students view knowledge. Knowledge becomes active, something that students experience in real-life situations. Learning becomes personal and affects how we react and respond in future situations.

Box 5.1 • Principles of Experiential Education Practice.

Principles of experiential education practice are

- Experiential learning occurs when carefully chosen experiences are supported by reflection, critical analysis, and synthesis.
- Experiences are structured to require the learner to take initiative, make decisions, and be accountable for results.
- Throughout the experiential process, the learner is actively engaged in posing questions, investigating, experimenting, being curious, solving problems, assuming responsibility, being creative, and constructing meaning.
- Learners are engaged intellectually, emotionally, socially, soulfully, and/or physically. This involvement produces a perception that the learning task is authentic.
- The results of learning are personal and form the basis for future experience and learning.
- Relationships are developed and nurtured: learner to self, learner to others, and learner to the world at large.
- The educator and learner may experience success, failure, adventure, risk-taking, and uncertainty, because the outcomes of the experience cannot totally be predicted.
- Opportunities are nurtured for learners and educators to explore and examine their own values.
- The educator's primary roles include setting suitable experiences, posing problems, setting boundaries, supporting learners, insuring physical and emotional safety, and facilitating the learning process.
- The educator recognizes and encourages spontaneous opportunities for learning.
- Educators strive to be aware of their biases, judgments, preconceptions, and how these influence the learner.
- The design of learning experience includes the possibility to learn from natural consequences, mistakes, and successes.

Source: Website of Association for Experiential Education. Available at: http://www.aee.org.

• Preceptor Pearls •

Utilization of the principles of experiential education can maximize the experiential experience for both preceptor and student.

As experiential educators in pharmacy practice, a preceptor's job is to engage students in real-life pharmacy activities with real consequences that allow students to achieve prescribed learning objectives. Often, we are co-experimenters with our students, not knowing ahead of time the outcome of the situations in which we involve them. At the end of the day, we must reflect on the learning activities we have designed and respond to students' reactions to these activities.[3,4]

• Preceptor Pearls •

"Real life" experiential experiences are vital to the growth and maturity of the student.

In an experiential learning environment, students must learn while doing. They must move beyond being knowledge gatherers, instead creating knowledge for themselves based on the real-life experiences and consequences in which they are actively involved. Students must also learn to respond to and reflect on their experiences and to take accountability for their actions.[3,4]

• Preceptor Pearls •

Reflection and discussion of these experiences are key for the continued improvement of future experiences.

Experiential education is the requisite step that transforms pharmacy students armed with basic facts and skills into mature pharmacy practitioners who are able to integrate and apply knowledge to solve problems and manage patient drug therapies. Perhaps more importantly, the model of experiential education that a student experiences during his or her education will shape how that student approaches the lifelong learning process necessary to continue to be a successful and competent pharmacy practitioner. By serving as the facilitator for experiential education activities within our practice setting we not only elevate our own knowledge level, but we also insure the future and vitality of our profession.

Learning Strategies for Preceptors and Students

The development of theories, taxonomies, ideologies, and studies about the way a person learns has led to the idea that students and educators alike should consider how the individual student learns in educational situations both in and outside of the classroom.[5] The idea that a one size lecture fits all may not be exactly right. In fact, educators should be as concerned with the way students learn as they are with the content of a course. The idea that individual learning styles are key to course development is, in part, responsible for a movement in the last 20 years in medical and pharmacy education toward more student centered activities. Curriculum in colleges of pharmacy have been adapted to include problem- or outcomes-based approaches to teaching as a result of overarching theories such as constructivism.[5]

Experiential education is also a model of learning and is based on theories of Kolb and others.[5] Both problem-based and outcomes oriented approaches and experiential education are methods for helping students to learn and to meet goals and objectives set by faculty. Curriculum in colleges of pharmacy, even individual courses that incorporate experiential education, should be designed using multiple types of teaching methods, and push students to use various levels of knowledge. Using this approach will allow individual students to learn in a manner that is comfortable for them. Recognizing that students do not all learn the same way or at the same pace will aid the preceptor in putting in place activities that meet curriculum objectives at the experiential education site. Preceptors should be concerned that their teaching helps the students' learn knowledge, skills and applications, and attitude. The following discussion provides a brief overview of Bloom's taxonomy, which is not a learning theory, such as constructivism or a model such as experiential education, but a naming structure for categorizing domains or areas of student learning.

After World War II, Bloom and associates, educational psychologists at the University of Chicago, developed what has become the most widely used taxonomy in education created, at the time, to assess students' learning. It categorizes learning into three psychological domains or ways of learning: cognitive, affective, and behavioral. Bloom never intended it for the categories of learning to be a theory or philosophy, but simply a means to assess student learning. However, over time, Bloom's taxonomy has come to be used as a way to both assess and define objective measures of learning for students. The overarching ideas of the acquisition of knowledge, skills, and attitudes, which build on learning theories, may help preceptors devise different activities for learning the same information for individual students.[6]

Preceptors ought to want to understand and employ the basics of this taxonomy when developing activities and objectives for a course, and creating activities for students. Cognitive and affective learning both describe the acquisition of knowledge, skills, or attitudes during the course of an individual experience (Table 5.1). Some student's perform better at the cognitive and affective level, but some students need to practice and apply information to learn, leading to the importance of the behavioral domain for experiential education. Bloom's taxonomy is structured as a hierarchy, beginning with lower-order thinking, or knowledge, and then moving up the scale to higher order, or evaluation. Students can actually learn in any order and should be encouraged to do so. As the discussion continues of cognitive versus affective learning, keep in mind the original intent of the taxonomy was not as learning theory; thus, some of the comments may appear to be an approach to assessment, but remember that in the context of this chapter, the domains are being used as means of learning.[6]

Table 5.1 • Taxonomy from Bloom, Krathwohl, and Masia[7]			
Cognitive Learning	Or	Affective Learning	Or
Knowledge	*Has data*	*Receiving*	*Accepts*
Comprehension	*Understands*	*Responding*	*Takes action*
Application	*Treats*	*Valuing*	*Respects*
Analysis	*Investigates*	*Organizing*	*Manages*
Synthesis	*Blends*	*Internalizing*	
Evaluation	*Appraises*		

Source: References 6, 8, and 9.

• Preceptor Pearls •

Using Bloom's taxonomy can help determine appropriateness of assignments.

Behavioral, or psychomotor as originally named, learning is important in the setting of experiential education. Behavioral learning implies the acquisition of skills and development of competence in performance of procedures, operations, methods, and techniques. In experiential education for pharmacy students, these could be the technical skills of making or dispensing an intravenous admixture. Behavioral learning can include simple motor tasks that students must learn to perform, but to move toward competence as a professional in the performance of procedures, methods, and techniques students must integrate knowledge learned. The preceptor may have to develop activities, which enable the student to practice that integration and achieve the desired outcome or objective.[10] In the area of patient care, at the highest level of behavioral learning is the skill of origination. Developing patient therapeutic plans, patient histories, and disease state management education are just a few examples of behavioral learning at the most complex level.[6,8,9]

• Preceptor Pearls •

Psychomotor learning is as important as cognitive and affective learning in an experiential education course.

Cognitive learning is the acquisition of knowledge and information. Multiple-choice questions effectively evaluate cognitive learning because they assess what facts students remember or have memorized for the examination. There is no guarantee that, at the most basic cognitive functioning level, students can incorporate these facts into anything useful.[6,8,9]

The hierarchy of affective learning involves the development of attitudes, feelings, and preferences.[6,8,9] However, it is difficult to assess receiving, responding, valuing, organizing, and internalizing of information by the learner. Enabling of this kind of learning by students can occur through development of professional presentations or of their ability to organize and relay information to others. The preceptor can assess the learning, through evaluation of these activities.

Introductory pharmacy practice experiences (IPPEs) and advanced pharmacy practice experiences (APPEs) require that students jump into tasks at a site, and the students may not have had much chance to learn some of the knowledge required. One analogy is to presume that students are empty computer disks, and it is the job of the teachers to help the students create files on the disk. In truth, it is not so simple because experiential education involves more than writing files to a disk. In other words, although facts are important, it is the concepts, application of knowledge, and desire to learn that will stay with students. Preceptors ought to recognize that individuals learn differently, at different paces, and that there are different domains of learning. It is up to the preceptor to determine the right blend of teachable moments and when it is appropriate to push for more active learning on the part of the student.

• Preceptor Pearls •

Not all students are on the same starting line; learning what the student already knows can improve their outcome in a course.

Student-Centered Learning vs. Teacher-Centered Learning

Teaching and learning often occur separately, despite a teacher's best efforts and teaching methods. Learning can occur during reading, writing, or reflection; both with or without a teacher; in groups or individually; and on purpose or by accident. It is often education that gets in the way of learning, for example, by making an assumption that the lecture format fits all student learning needs, or that every student learns what they need in a group setting. Student- and teacher-centered learning methods dictate that learning revolves either around the students or around what the teacher believes students should learn.

Many people in faculty roles today learned the teacher-centered model of education. In this passive approach to learning, the teacher stands in the front of the classroom and presents information to fill the blank computer disks in students' heads. When this occurs, students have little time to file the information in a format in which they can easily retrieve it for later use. Students may hear every word the professor says, and they may even manage to write everything down on paper. However, neither of these actions requires that students process the information, and students are passive learners (if they learn at all). A student-centered approach to learning may be far more successful.

• Preceptor Pearls •

Learning is not a passive activity.

The educational reform that moved the focus to the student began in 1997 with the American Psychological Association.[10] In this approach the teacher does not necessarily stand up in front of a class or decide exactly which information to teach students or how he or she will teach it. Rather, the approach requires active involvement of students because when they are engaged, they are more likely learn (Table 5.2).[6,7,11,12] Under ideal conditions, students will learn if they are actively involved and if what they are learning affects their inner selves. Students have to find the information personally important. In the classroom or even on experiential education courses, students often do not learn what a faculty member thinks they should learn because they do not sense the importance.[6]

• Preceptor Pearls •

Adopting a student-centered learning approach improves your experiential education program.

In order to promote learning, preceptors must be authentic and accepting of students as individuals who bring value to the activities at the site. Many colleges or schools of pharmacy require

Table 5.2 • Comparison of Instructional Styles	
Teacher-Centered Activities	**Student-Centered Activities**
Passive	*Active*
Rewards students who can memorize well but not transfer data to other applications	*Rewards researchers, questioners, and problem solvers*
	Small group discussions
Primary responsibility to relay data to a group	*Group projects*
Communication, one way (i.e., lecture)	*Reflective activities*
Questioning	*Peer teaching*
Demonstration	*Role playing*
Source: References 11 and 13.	

that students send a résumé or curriculum vitae before attendance at a site. These documents help faculty members and preceptors understand student accomplishments and their level of prior learning. A preceptor should review these documents prior to meeting with the student the first time. It is important to promote what students know and to facilitate their learning based on that. During curriculum vitae review a preceptor may help students find a new perspective or insight into the information they have already learned, and gather thoughts about what they need to learn. Remember that faculty and preceptors must be able to relate to students on some level in order to have an impact on the learning.[14]

These ideal conditions may seem too difficult to achieve in a setting in which the primary responsibility of preceptors is to do their job as pharmacists as opposed to teaching students. There are ways to accomplish both tasks effectively and perhaps improve performance at all levels. A good teacher will learn from his or her students. It is not enough to just engage students in activities and expect them to learn. Learners need support, guidance, and a chance to reflect on what they know and what they need to know. With that said, it is not always the responsibility of the preceptor to provide this for students. Students often do well when involved in groups with their peers. They learn in groups because they have the opportunity to brainstorm; to present ideas; and to have ideas evaluated, rejected or remodeled, and improved. Small groups increase the commitment of each student. Students have changes in attitudes and behaviors when they work in small groups. In some cases, small groups may not affect cognitive learning, but they do impact affective learning.[14] Assigning students to groups and creating learning communities among students also relieves the preceptor from always providing the opportunities for teaching, reflecting, and learning.

This student-centered approach may initially cause challenges to preceptors. If students have never been exposed to this method, they will not immediately know how to act, may appear not to be learning, and may be defensive in their new role. There are several activities that a preceptor can use to get students used to active learning, beginning with individual activities and moving on to group activities. Writing is a common and effective method for learning. When students engage in writing by answering directed questions or in free-flow discussion of a topic, they write what they know and they learn what they do not. Students often initially rebel against free-flow discussion and writing, but many will learn that reflection helps them.

The EXPLORE (examine, pair, listen, organize, research, and evaluate) process is another way to encourage constructive learning. Instructors first present students with a controversial statement and ask them to commit themselves to a position relating to the issue. The instructors then pair two students who are on opposing sides of the controversy. Each person listens to the other's view so he or she can summarize it accurately. Once hearing each other's point of view, the students put the arguments into a compare-and-contrast table. Then they research the issue to find supporting literature about either side. The pair then compares their findings and agrees on research-based statements.[15] Employing either of these techniques will help students become actively engaged in their learning.

• Preceptor Pearls •

The teachable moment becomes an "ah-ha" moment when students are engaged.

One quality measure that a preceptor may use to evaluate individual and group learning is to get input. Pierce has suggested that if students do not view an assignment as appropriate, instructors should allow them to identify and create an alternative assignment that will meet the same outcomes.[15] This will likely require patience and direction by the preceptor. At the end of the experiential education course students should reflect on assignments and the amount and value of the learning from each activity. If the assignment was not helpful in learning, students should say so and support their opinions with examples or suggestions.[15] This activity provides the faculty or preceptor with feedback on activities and provides suggestions for replacements that may provide improved benefit to students.

Choosing student-centered learning over teacher-centered teaching can provide a conundrum for preceptors and faculty with busy schedules, lack of experience, and too many things on the to-do list. Preceptors and faculty rely heavily on the teacher-centered method of teaching simply because it may not pose as many difficulties, or obstacles, as the student-centered approach. Teachers who lecture and are only concerned with knowledge may not be put on the spot with questions. They are able to control the direction of lectures. When using the student-centered approach, teachers can encourage students to ask questions, which may change the direction of the lecture. Preceptors using the student-centered approach must be able to adapt and move with the learning, even if it feels as if he or she has lost all control of the topic to the students.[16] Many students make it to their experiential education courses and have not yet learned how to learn. It is these students who may pose the most difficulty for preceptors when employing methods that encourage student-centered learning. These few tricky situations may cause a bit of unease at first, not only for preceptors but also for the students as they learn how to learn. Moving in the direction of adding more student-centered learning activities may be a delightful, if unexpected, adventure in learning for both the preceptor and the student.[16]

Students report more enjoyable learning experiences and changes in attitudes with the student-centered approach.[11] Table 5.3 matches Bloom's domains with methods or models of instruction that help students achieve and learn. It is important for both full-time faculty and the many adjunct professors and preceptors to recognize Bloom's taxonomy when evaluating what students have learned and to develop a method of teaching that recognizes that not all students are alike when it comes to learning. If students are to learn to think like pharmacists, to be problem-solvers, and to become lifelong learners then they must learn to reflect, evaluate, validate, and verify. These skills are not inherent—students must learn how to learn, and teachers and preceptors can help them.

Table 5.3 • Matching Domain and Level of Learning to Appropriate Methods

Domain and Level of Learning from Bloom's Taxonomy	Method
COGNITIVE	
Knowledge	*Lecture, programmed instruction, drill, and practice*
Comprehension	*Lecture, programmed instruction*
Application	*Discussion, simulation and games, field experience, laboratory*
Analysis	*Discussion, independent/group projects, simulations, field experience, role playing, laboratory*
Synthesis	*Independent/group projects, field experience, role playing, laboratory*
Evaluation	*Independent/group projects, field experience, role playing, laboratory*
AFFECTIVE	
Receiving	*Lecture, discussion, field experience*
Responding	*Discussion, simulations, role playing, field experience*
Valuing	*Discussion, independent/group projects, simulations, role playing, field experience*
Organization	*Discussion, independent/group projects, field experience*

Source: Reference 11.

Developing Lifelong Learning Habits

Lifelong learning includes "all learning activity undertaken throughout life, with the aim of improving knowledge, skills, and competences within a personal, civic, social, and/or employment-related perspective."[17] As a preceptor you have the unique opportunity to affect not only the professional development but also the lifelong learning habits of the students with whom you come in contact in any situation. It is through your personal development, actions, and comments that these young professionals will begin the development of their own thoughts and ideas around lifelong learning habits. Therefore it is of extreme importance that preceptors recognize the vigilant observations of the students they precept.

With the advent of new Accreditation Council on Pharmacy Education (ACPE) standards as they pertain to pharmacy practice experiences, a greater number of pharmacy students will be spending time earlier in their pharmacy education in a multitude of pharmacy settings to meet the required hours for introductory pharmacy practice experiences (IPPEs). The IPPEs, while providing the students with exposure to a variety of practice settings, will provide students the opportunity to begin forming lifelong learning habits. Practice settings expose students to the professionalism and educational standards by which practicing pharmacists engage in real-life pharmacy jobs.

The role that academicians play in the pharmacy students' future is of vital importance, but it is through the engagement of preceptors and their fellow colleagues that these students will begin to form their own opinions and personal practices for the development of lifelong learning habits. Lifelong learning habits must engage pharmacy practitioners in more than the minimal continuing education requirements currently in place by state boards of pharmacy. Continuing education sessions (live, web-based, recorded, written production, etc.) are not the most appropriate means by which lifelong learning and personal improvement brings about better outcomes for patients.

• Preceptor Pearls •

Development of lifelong learning habits are key to providing our patients with the highest level of care.

Continuous professional development (CPD) is "an ongoing, self-directed, structured, outcomes-focused cycle of learning and personal improvement."[17] Such organizations as ACPE, the Chartered Institute of Personnel and Development (CIPD), and *Fédération Internationale Pharmaceutique* (International Pharmaceutical Federation, or FIP) reference and define CPD. They discuss the theme of self-directed, ongoing, structured learning and building of one's knowledge, skills, and attitudes that are necessary to ensure competence in one's given profession. The process of CPD helps provide pharmacists with the resources to provide patients with the best care possible.

• Preceptor Pearls •

Continuous professional development is an excellent tool for a practitioner to utilize at any point in his or her career.

The concept of CPD involves practitioners' reflecting personally on their practice to assess their knowledge and skills, to identify deficits or needs, to formulate an individualized learning plan of action, to and assess the effectiveness of their educational interventions and their plan of action as it pertains to their practice. An extremely important piece of CPD is documentation, which makes a personal portfolio a key component.[17] Pharmacy experiential educators are requiring that pharmacy students begin this journey of lifelong learning by forming their own portfolio and following this method of CPD. Simply put, CPD is planning, acting, evaluating, reflecting, and keeping the record (the portfolio) of these activities.

While CPD is a means by which many schools of pharmacy are preparing their students to become lifelong learners, it is ultimately up to the individuals to continue to pursue these endeavors. It is critically important that the pharmacy students you precept see that you lead by example. Your own CPD and your discussion of the pharmacy students' CPD will provide a firm foundation on which the pharmacy student can and will succeed both professionally as well as personally. It is through this process that both current and future practitioners will be able to help people make the best use of medicines and thus provide them with the best possible outcomes.

• Preceptor Pearls •

Preceptors are in a key role to lead by example and provide an firm foundation on which students will continue to build their own educational foundations throughout their careers.

Developing Workplace Skills

Workplace skills are just as important to pharmacy students as their academic knowledge. Workplace skills are those skills required in employees to be successful in their career. They are the nonacademic characteristics that determine professionalism and lead to job success. During the 1990s there was an increased focus by the business community to identify and correct deficiencies in the preparation of students of the workforce. In 1991, The U.S. Department of Labor presented a report of the Secretary's Commission on Achieving Necessary Skills (SCANS report) in which a minimum set of workplace skills were noted.[18,19] The report identified five SCAN competencies considered critical in today's workforce and include (1) resources (2) interpersonal (3) information (4) systems and (5) technology.[18,19] The optimal place for pharmacy students to develop these workplace skills is outside of the confines of the classroom and in the real world setting provided by pharmacy practice apprenticeship experiences under the preceptor's guidance.[19,20]

Resources refer to the ability to identify, organize, plan, and allocate resources.[18] By the time they reach their practice experiences most students have only had the opportunity to utilize these skills on themselves. Full understanding of this process comes from having the experience of having to plan for resources and then having to adjust the plan as needed.

To help students develop their resource skills, allow the students to participate in the following:

- Allow the students to create a schedule for the activities of the day including workflow, meetings, etc. Then allow for the emergencies (fire drills, critical patient needs, etc.) to slip in. This will allow the students the opportunity to prioritize and also realize that sometimes the work is not finished in an 8-hour day.

- Present all projects required for the practice experience to the students at the onset of the practice experience. Allow the students to set the due dates for the project, but do not allow for adjustments to the timetables. This will also give the students a broader understanding of the importance of deadlines and managing projects and resources through to deadlines in situations where there is competition for time.

- Allow the students to work with a portion of the pharmacy budget. Provide them with an understanding of the daily, weekly, monthly, and annual pharmacy budget constraints with regard to purchasing. Have them work with the pharmacy buyer to determine ways to stay within the budget. Provide them also with case scenarios in which a specific patient (resistance, multiple complications, factor deficiencies, etc.) can cause a budget crisis and ask them what changes they would make to the budget because of this situation.

- Allow them to work with your department scheduler to make an upcoming staff schedule. Provide them with opportunities to make recommendations on how to appropriately staff vacations, holidays, or staffing shortages. Ask the students to prioritize the different roles in the pharmacy department to validate their knowledge of the impact of the different roles.

- Discuss with the students the importance of skills assessment or competency validation. Ask the students to participate the in the creation and validation of a specific competency.

The interpersonal workplace skill competency deals with the students' ability to function as a part of a team.[18] However, this competency is more complex than just functioning as a member of the team, it also involves serving as a leader of a team, negotiating for results or conflict resolution, and working with diversity.

To help the students learn more about cooperation and teamwork, the students should be given the opportunity to do the following:

- Work as a member of a particular team (examples include the pharmacy team, a medication safety team, a medical rounding team, etc.).

- Lead a team to find a solution to a common problem (work-up a patient for rounds, prepare an agenda for and lead a meeting).

- Work with teams that are made up of different types of people (patients, nurses, physicians, or other healthcare providers).

- Work with patients and colleagues of different ethnic, cultural, educational, and economic backgrounds.

- Work in a small, controlled group, and assume different roles in the group (leader, devil's advocate, etc.).

While the students are having these experiences have dialogue with the students about what preparation should be done proactively to prepare for the meetings. Help the students to frame and understand the audience participating in the meetings. After the meeting discuss with the students their participation in the meeting including (1) Did the students play a role in the meeting, (2) What was the intended outcome of the meeting, (3) What was the actual outcome of the meeting, (4) What could have been done better, and (5) Did anyone bring with them baggage from outside of the meeting that influenced the meeting and how could that have been avoided? Having these types of conversations with the students not only provides them with the ability to analyze and understand teams, but also teaches them to do some basic environmental scanning. Finally, in reviewing this you are teaching the students to go back and assess their meeting, team, and success. This practice of assessing and adjusting will also be another workplace skill that the students can take with them.

The next competency is probably one of the easiest and most difficult today. The information competency or that ability to acquire and evaluate information is very important.[18] We are living in the day and age of rapid access knowledge. Never have we lived in a time where knowledge is more abundant. There is instantaneous access to information on any topic from your computer, GPS, iPod, or even your mobile phone.

The challenge with this abundance of knowledge is twofold. The first challenge is assessing the validity of the information. The students must have the understanding that not all of the information available to them is accurate. The preceptor can work with the students to help them validate reliable sources for information and identify inappropriate sources of information. The next challenge is that of how to use the information. A preceptor can work with the students to determine how the students organize, interpret, and process the information. Examples of ways to work with the students on this include the following:

- Journal article review and comparison to nonprimary literature
- Medication evaluation of an herbal product where there is limited primary literature but an abundance of Internet information
- Medication histories from the patient, from a family member and from the patient's pharmacy, to compare the difference in the reliability of the information

Any deficiencies in the aforementioned areas provide an opportunity for the preceptor to work with the students to develop these skills.

The fourth competency focuses on systems and specifically the understanding of complex relationships and interrelationships.[18] The first aspect of this is helping the students to understand how organizational, social, and technology systems work together. After exposure to how these systems work together, the next step involves helping the students to understand the monitoring and adjustment of the systems performance. Students should be trained to assess the systems and make recommendations for improvements. This assessment and feedback loop should be a continuous process that students hardwire into their skill set.

Examples of how students can understand the interrelationship include the following:

- Allow students to map out the medication-use process in your facility or practice site. Have them identify the key stakeholders in the medication-use process. Allow them the opportunity to discuss what would happen if any of these stakeholders were not able to perform.
- Work with the students to understand the continuum of care for the patient, from the moment an order is written in a hospital, through the patient's discharge, to management in the ambulatory setting. Ask the students to identify the patient specific needs associated with the continuum including outcomes, financial needs, and social needs of the patient.

The final competency refers to technology and the ability of the students to be able to utilize a wide variety of technologies.[18] The students should be able to appropriately select the type of technology they need to accomplish a task, apply the selected technology to accomplish the desired outcomes, and troubleshoot malfunctions of the technology. The world of pharmacy is full of technology including procurement systems, order-entry software, automation, and robotics to name just a few. Early and frequent exposure to these different types of technology allow the students to gain a better understanding of the types of technology available, the current breath of technology, the variations between products, and the future of technology. Allowing the students to have controlled exposure to the types of technology and how they interact will be a foundation for competency in technology. Examples of technology to expose the students to include

- Pharmacy automation systems
- Pharmacy order-entry systems
- Clinical pharmacy information systems and databases
- The latest glucometers or other point of service devices

- Laboratory technology, including technology that calculates and records laboratory values and cultures and sensitivities

Competencies in (1) resources, (2) interpersonal, (3) information, (4) systems, and (5) technology are critical workplace skills.[18-20] However, the ability to develop and adapt these skills is not something that can be taught from a book; they are all experience driven. Pharmacy practice experiences provide preceptors the opportunity to provide the foundations of these competencies to the students before they enter the workforce. As a practice experience is planned, taking advantage of opportunities to maximize exposure to these competencies is critical for development of future pharmacists with good workplace skills.

Summary

Experiential teaching is the life blood of the academic process for creating pharmacy professionals from the foundation of pharmacy students. APPEs may be defined as the culmination of 3 professional years of didactic work as well as a minimally required amount of IPPEs. It is through both IPPEs and APPEs that pharmacy students are influenced, molded, and begin to take their very own shape as pharmacy professionals. Thus, these experiences are key to "putting all the pieces together" and creating the students' reality of the practice of pharmacy. It is important for both preceptors and students to find the most productive learning approach for all individuals involved. The installation of lifelong learning habits is a crucial component of the continuous professional development of any practitioner and is vital to the experiential teaching process. It is vital for all preceptors to understand their role as a professional mentor to all students they may come in contact with, in as well as outside of the walls of their pharmacy. Development of workplace skills is yet another essential factor to the experiences that students should take away from their experiential teaching and may influence them throughout their career. These key aspects of experiential teaching will assist both you and your students in making the most of their experiential teachings both now and in the future. Remember, it is the influence of these essential learning experiences, good or bad, that will mold future careers and the profession of pharmacy.

References

1. Association of Experiential Education. Principles of Experiential Education Practice. Available at: http://www.aee.org/customer/pages.php?pageid=47. Accessed June 14, 2008.

2. Accreditation Council for Pharmacy Education. *Accreditation Standards and Guidelines for the Professional Program in Pharmacy Leading to the Doctor of Pharmacy Degree.* Chicago, IL: Accreditation Council for Pharmacy Education; 2007.

3. Itin CM. Reasserting the philosophy of experiential education as a vehicle for change in the 21st century. *J Exp Edu.* 1999;22:91-8.

4. Wikipedia. Experiential Education. Available at: *http://en.wikipedia.org/wiki/Experiential_education.* Accessed June 14, 2008.

5. Learning Theories Knowledgebase (November 2008). Index of Learning Theories and Models at Learning-Theories.com. Available at: http://www.learningtheories.com. Accessed November 30, 2008.

6. Shulman L. Making differences: a table of learning. *Change.* 2002;Nov/Dec:36–44.

7. Schwartz W. Education in the classroom. *J High Educ.* 1980;51:235–54.

8. Lopez C. Opportunities for Improvement: Advice from Consultant-Evaluators on Programs to Assess Student Learning. Chicago, IL: North Central Association of Colleges and Schools; March 1996 (reprinted April 1997). ERIC Document Reproduction Service No. ED 463 790.

9. Leith, K. Adult learning styles and the college classroom. Paper presented at: Annual Meeting of the American Psychological Association; August 22–25, 2002; Chicago. EDRS Document Reproduction Service No. ED470 010 CG 032 020.

10. Dembo H. Don't lose sight of the students. *Princip Leadership.* 2004;4:37–42.

11. Weston C, Cranton P. Selecting instructional strategies. *J High Educ.* 1986;57:259–83.

12. Spencer J, Jordan R. Learner centered approaches in medical education. *Br Med J.* 1999;518:1280–3.

13. Kopp S, Seestedt-Stanford L, Rohlfing K, et al. Creating adaptive environments. *Planning Higher Ed.* 2004;32:12–23.

14. Barbour A. Group Methods and Affective Learning. Report No. CS 509 927. Denver, CO: University of Denver School of Communications; 1998. ERIC Document Reproduction Service No. ED 424 599.

15. Pierce J, Kalkman D. Applying learner-centered principles in teacher education. *Theory Into Prac.* 2003;(42)2:127–32.

16. Zophy, J. On learner-centered teaching. *The History Teacher.* 1982;15(2):185–96. The Scholarly Journal Archive (JSTOR). Available at: www.jstor.org.novacat.nova.edu/jstore/gifcvtdir/ap001332/00182745. Accessed May 5, 2008.

17. Rouse MJ. Continuing professional development in pharmacy. *Am J Health Syst Pharm.* 2004;61:2069–76.

18. US Department of Labor. The Secretary's Commission on Achieving Necessary Skills (1991). What Work Requires of Schools. A SCANS report for America 2000. Washington, DC: US Government Printing Office.

19. Holter NC, Kopka DJ. Developing a workplace skills course: lessons learned. *J Edu Bus.* 2001;Jan:138–43.

20. Lerman, RI. Building a wider skills net for workers. *Issues Sci Technol.* 2008;summer:65–72.

Example is the school of mankind, and they will learn at no other.
Kurt Herbert Alder

Chapter 6

Fundamentals of Experiential Teaching

Jordan F. Dow, Lee C. Vermeulen, Linda Stevens Albrecht, Kristen Mizgate Bader, Todd W. Canada, Tammy Cohen, Diane B. Ginsburg, Molly E. Graham, Grace M. Kuo, Michael Piñón, Ruth E. Nemire, Dehuti A. Pandya, Kevin Purcell, Margie E. Snyder

Chapter Outline

Learning Objectives

- Describe introductory pharmacy practice experiences and discuss appropriate learning opportunities for introductory practice experience students.

- Express important considerations when preparing for and precepting an introductory experience student.

- Provide examples of the usefulness and importance of intermediate experiences.

- Review common principles that guide advanced experiential education.

- Describe professional and interpersonal skills relating to the practice of pharmacy in an interdisciplinary environment.

- Identify the different types of learners and become familiar with what teaching techniques are effective for each type.

- Explain the logic-based method of teaching.

- Explain the importance of providing ongoing feedback to students in pharmacy practice experiences.

- Describe the use of the summative evaluation methods to evaluate students in pharmacy practice experiences.

- Identify factors in the practice setting that may contribute to student difficulty.

- Identify strategies for dealing with a difficult student and/or situation.

- Outline an approach for designing a program curriculum and constructing a program manual.

- Provide ideas for creating an intern practice model and involving others in experiential training.

- Discuss methods for evaluating the effectiveness and success of a program.

- Describe key components of continuous quality improvement in an experiential education program.

Experiential teaching has its rewards and its frustrations. In all, being a preceptor is well worth the sacrifice of time and energy to teach and develop the next generation of pharmacists. This chapter is designed to help you become an effective experiential teacher. The chapter begins with a review of the practice experiences that pharmacy students complete. From there, it reveals the necessary techniques for reaching different types of students, and how to handle precepting challenges. Finally, the chapter provides a guide for developing and implementing an experiential learning program and discloses how to continually assess and improve the quality of your program.

Introductory Practice Experiences

Historically, pharmacy education separated didactic, classroom instruction and site-based experiential rotations. The typical pharmacy curriculum was segmented with the first 3 years devoted to classroom instruction and labs, and with the fourth year dedicated to experiential rotations. Some students gained site-based experience during their first 3 years of school through summer internships or other pharmacy work experience, but there was no formal connection between the experiences and the pharmacy curriculum. The absence of integrated classroom teaching and experiential training during the first 3 years of pharmacy school resulted in many students struggling through their transition from the classroom to the required fourth-year experiential rotations, now known as advanced pharmacy practice experiences (APPEs).

Recognizing this educational gap, the Accreditation Council for Pharmacy Education (ACPE) adopted new curricular standards for the Doctor of Pharmacy (Pharm.D.) program.[1] These standards went into effect in July 2007. An important part of the new standards is the requirement of introductory pharmacy practice experiences (IPPEs). These introductory experiences are hands-on opportunities for pharmacy students to gain experience in a variety of practice settings early in their education. The purposes of the introductory experiences are to enable students to apply some of the knowledge they are acquiring in their didactic courses, to prepare pharmacy students for their advanced practice experiences that they will complete during their final year of pharmacy school, and to expose pharmacy students to actual pharmacy practice sites. The introductory practice experiences are scheduled during the first, second, and third professional years of the Pharm.D. curriculum and are designed to complement material taught in the students' Pharm.D. courses.

The updated ACPE standards state that IPPEs should make up 5% of the total Pharm.D. curriculum.[1] This equals approximately 300 hours of practice experience that are to be distributed over the first 3 years of students' education. To ensure that students meet their learning objectives, these experiences are distinct from pharmacy summer internships or other shadowing experiences students may have pursued on their own. IPPEs are applied toward course credit, along with graduation and professional licensure requirements, so students may not receive remuneration for their time.

Schools may offer introductory practice experiences in many areas of pharmacy practice, but at minimum students are required to complete experiences in community and hospital pharmacy settings. Many schools have students engage in shadowing or service learning exercises during their early years, but the schools will only recognize these activities as introductory practice experiences if they afford students the opportunity to develop specific patient care skills. Experiences that only focus on the development of students' professionalism or leadership abilities are not considered introductory practice experiences.

Students will have many learning opportunities during their community and hospital introductory practice experiences. In both settings students should learn the following fundamental skills:

- Basic pharmacy management principles
- Prescription/order processing and compounding
- Adverse drug event reporting
- Drug information skills

- Medication safety
- Development of a drug-related problem list
- Protection of patient privacy and confidentiality
- Patient assessment and pharmacotherapy
- Patient interview skills including allergy information
- Patient education skills
- Interprofessional communication skills
- Ethical behavior and empathy toward patients

In states that allow formal collaborative practice agreements, students may also have the opportunity to observe preceptors performing disease management activities. In the community setting, students may assist patients with over-the-counter medication selections, identify noncompliance or medication affordability concerns, and participate in the development of medication therapy management services or community outreach events. In the hospital, students may assist with medication safety initiatives, medical and nursing education, bedside and discharge patient education, medical patient care rounds, medication reconciliation services, other ongoing medication management or drug monitoring programs, and the development of new clinical programs.

A number of strategies have been used successfully to teach patient care skills and engage students in a meaningful way during their experiential rotations. Partnering fourth-year advanced practice students with students completing introductory experiences is one method.[2] This partnership improved introductory students' self-perceived patient care abilities and resulted in a smaller time commitment by faculty preceptors.[2] The partnership teaching method was studied and found to be effective across multiple practice sites, including hospital and outpatient environments; therefore, preceptors from varying backgrounds could consider this approach in the training they provide pharmacist interns. This partnership method of teaching could be further enhanced by including pharmacist residents in the learning experience. Utilizing preceptors from other professional backgrounds (i.e., physicians and nurse practitioners) has also been shown to be effective.[3] This approach fosters the development of collaborative relationships and an opportunity for students to better understand both the pharmacist role and the role of other healthcare workers in providing patient care. Focusing on the development of specific patient care skills has also been an effective student engagement strategy. For example, some students have had the opportunity to provide immunizations during their introductory experiences.[4] In states that allow this, administering immunizations provides pharmacist interns unique opportunities to gain confidence in both administration technique and communication with patients. By offering unique introductory experiences, preceptors can help students build confidence in their patient care skills while benefiting from the students' contributions to the preceptor's practice.

A few considerations are warranted when precepting introductory students. First, recognize that students completing an introductory experience are earlier in their education than fourth-year students, so their pharmacy knowledge base is substantially smaller. This does not mean that you should have lower expectations of introductory students than those of advanced students, but they must be different. The expectations must be in line with how far students have progressed within the professional sequence. Also, because introductory students have less classroom education, they may require more direction and supervision than fourth-year students. This potential burden can be minimized by using the multiple techniques discussed above. On the positive side, introductory experiences are commonly pharmacy students' first look into actual pharmacy practice. These early experiences are an exciting time for pharmacy students and it can be fun for preceptors to be a part of the experiences, guiding students and helping them gain an understanding of pharmacy practice. Students are very impressionable at this stage in their career, so preceptors play a key role in shaping student views of pharmacy practice. Considering this, take care to ensure introductory students have a positive experience. Lastly, introductory students are early in their pharmacy curriculum and tend to be excited to receive on-site training; they are typically motivated and eager to learn.

• Preceptor Pearls •

Make sure your expectations of introductory students are appropriate to their knowledge and skill levels.

Preceptors can prepare for introductory practice experiences in a number of ways. Prior to a student's scheduled learning experience, work with the course coordinator or experiential program director to ensure that you receive course learning objectives, a description of the methods used for student assessment, and a summary of concurrent didactic material taught in the Pharm.D. curriculum. Additionally, you may request guidance on appropriate methods for providing feedback to students. You may also inquire about the student you will be precepting in order to learn the professional level (e.g., second year, spring semester) and specific student strengths and areas of deficiency that the experience can address. This information may assist you in starting out on the same page as their students.

IPPEs are an important new addition to the Pharm.D. curriculum and will serve to enhance classroom learning and prepare students for APPEs. Preceptors have the opportunity to model essential patient care skills and significantly contribute to the professional development of introductory practice experience students.

Intermediate Practice Experiences

Back in pharmacy school, our family and friends inevitably called for medical advice, but early in our pharmacy education, those questions were likely difficult to answer. However, as our careers have progressed, those calls seem to get easier to handle. The professional experiences we've had influence the difference between our ability to aptly handle the calls we received during school and our ability to handle the calls we receive later in our careers. These professional experiences are invaluable, and the more experiences pharmacy students have, the stronger their foundation becomes and the greater the chance they have to grow and build on what they have learned.

The profession of pharmacy is built on lifelong learning, which starts early in one's career. The primary beginnings of this learning are through pharmacy practice experiences. The ACPE categorizes practice experiences into two sections. All experiences up until the final year of school are introductory experiences and all rotation experiences during the last year of school are categorized as advanced experiences.[1] This chapter is designed to show that learning experiences are a continuum. This section proposes a middle step between introductory and advanced experiences, namely intermediate experiences.

Intermediate experiences are not defined by ACPE, but they are the logical progression from the initial practice experiences to the advanced experiences. For example, a student may learn the structure and format of a patient chart during an initial experience, and then participate in data collection during an intermediate experience, and then work with the preceptor to analyze the data and come up with recommendations during an advanced experience. Exposing the student to various aspects of pharmacy over time allows him or her to assimilate the practicality of information, and it firmly engages him or her in pharmacy practice. Considering the student's previous experiences is critical in determining what tasks and responsibilities you should afford him or her.

Preceptors would likely agree that students who have a broad practical knowledge of pharmacy are more successful on rotations. One common complaint among specialized clinical practice preceptors is that students enter their rotations without basic practical clinical knowledge. For example, a student who only has experience in the retail setting would lack a foundation of hospital experience or general medicine experience. Without this experience, if the student is assigned to an ICU rotation on the first day of rotations, the ICU rotation will ultimately become a general hospital rotation or an internal medicine rotation despite the efforts of both the student and the preceptor. However, it is impractical for all students to be assigned first to a general hospital rotation. This example highlights the importance of having students complete intermediate rotations in various settings, so they can both gain experience and determine which type of fourth-year rotations they'd like to pursue.

• Preceptor Pearls •

Encourage an introductory student to pursue intermediate experiences to gain valuable experience and to determine career interest.

Intermediate experiences can include experiences outside of school oversight as well. Work internships are probably the best examples of this. They provide two key opportunities: first is exposure and second is marketability. Work internships allow students to try out pharmacy practice in various settings without an extensive time commitment. For example, students that have worked in a retail setting can take an internship at a hospital for the summer to gain exposure to the different practice settings and vice versa. Work internship commitments typically occur during the summer, so they give students insight into what practice would be like in the chosen settings, without committing students to that work setting long term. Students that complete a work internship can use that intermediate experience to guide their fourth-year rotation decisions, furthering them on their career path. For example, a student who completes a work internship in a hospital may find that he or she wants to pursue pharmacotherapy related to psychiatry. The student could use that information to choose multiple inpatient neurology or psychiatry-related rotations (as the program allows).

Besides exposure/experience, work internships offer marketability. Students who complete work internships have broader experience than those who do not complete them, and the work internship might have helped the students choose their desired area of practice based on their experiences. Potential employers, including employers who hire pharmacy residents, are excited about students who have had work internship experience.

Intermediate experiences are a means for today's pharmacy students to deepen their practical knowledge and to prepare themselves for the days of practicing on their own. The experiences provide an important step in the experiential training pathway, spanning and supplementing the gap between early introductory rotations and advanced experiences. Students commonly feel excitement, relief, and fear after passing the boards and realizing they can officially practice alone. The thoughts that they are now the final check, the last one to approve a medication, and the last opportunity to catch an error can make that transition period a difficult time. However, a solid didactic education combined with all of the hands-on knowledge acquired along the way can give confidence to a novice practitioner.

• Preceptor Pearls •

Familiarize yourself with your student's intermediate experiences.

Advanced Experiential Education

APPEs build on a solid foundation of IPPEs and extend into more focused areas of expertise (Box 6.1). There are many different areas in which pharmacists can become experts (Box 6.2); however, rather than discussing each area, this section aims to review common underlying principles that guide APPEs.

Box 6.1 • Advanced Experiential Education Goals

- To develop skills and competency in the advanced pharmacy practice areas of acute patient care, drug information and drug use policy development, ambulatory patient care, and health-system pharmacy management
- To provide a program designed to enhance student proficiency in providing a higher level of pharmacist care, developed from required, selective, and elective rotations
- To refine the teaching skills of preceptors in both the didactic and experiential training of students
- To provide a foundation for further training in a pharmacy practice (postgraduate year (PGY)-1 residency, specialized (PGY-2) residency or fellowship

Box 6.2 • Examples of Advanced Experiential Rotations

- Cardiology
- Critical care
- Clinical research
- Clinical toxicology
- Community pharmaceutical care
- Drug information/investigational drug services
- Emergency medicine
- General/trauma surgery
- Geriatrics
- Hospice or palliative care
- Infectious disease
- Medication safety
- Nephrology
- Neurosurgery or neurology
- Nutrition support
- OB/maternal/child
- Oncology
- Pediatrics
- Pharmacoeconomics
- Pharmacy informatics
- Primary/ambulatory care
- Psychiatry
- Pulmonology
- Transplantation
- Women's health

There are two main categories of skills that are considered to be fundamental to the practice of clinical pharmacy: professional and interpersonal, each with its own set of skills.

Professional Skills

Advanced practice experiences provide opportunities to develop and enhance a student's professional skills. Box 6.3 lists general activities that can help to refine those professional skills. Activities associated with specific skills appear below.

Box 6.3 • Examples of Student Activities on Advanced Experiential Rotations

- Formal patient case presentations
- Journal club presentations including reviews of pertinent articles for pharmacists
- Formal written drug information responses
- Pharmacy and therapeutics drug monographs
- Medwatch adverse event reports
- Formal in-service presentations regarding new treatments
- Topic discussions
- Formal research or writing projects
- Patient specific monitoring and evaluation
- Health promotion/disease prevention fair
- Grand rounds (medical or pharmacy)

Box 6.4 • Unique Experiential Experiences

- *Pediatric Camps: Diabetic, Hematology/Oncology, Hemophilia, Dialysis*

  Allows students to work in an interdisciplinary environment, advising and managing pediatric patients with chronic disease over a 1- or 6-week time period

- *American Association of Colleges of Pharmacy (AACP)*

  National organization that represents the interests of pharmaceutical education and educators; Alexandria, VA

- *American Pharmaceutical Association*

  Experiences in national association activities and operations, pharmacy practice issues, educational programming, state services, scientific affairs, student affairs, public relations, and project management; Washington, DC

- *American Society of Consultant Pharmacists*

  Provides students with experience and training in federal and state legislative and regulatory processes; focuses on pharmacy, long-term care, and other current healthcare issues being considered by federal and state legislative and regulatory bodies; Alexandria, VA

- *American Society of Health-System Pharmacists*

  Experiences in association activities and operations, publications and drug information systems, membership and organizational affairs, governmental affairs, professional and public affairs, student affairs, marketing, and product development; Bethesda, MD

Box 6.4 • Unique Experiential Experiences (cont'd)

- *Drug Topics*

  Provides experience in medical writing and drug information gathering; a 6-week program; Montvale, NJ

- *International Pharmacy Student Federation (IPSF)*

  Promotes interaction among pharmacists internationally in order to improve public health; many international experiential opportunities

- *National Naval Medical Center*

  Located on the National Naval Medical Command campus; convenient to numerous educational opportunities such as the National Cancer Institute (NCI) and the Henry M. Jackson Foundation for HIV/AIDS research; as a major teaching site for Navy healthcare professionals, numerous opportunities exist to interact on all academic and interdisciplinary levels; Bethesda, MD

- *United States Pharmacopeia*

  Develops standards for quality of medicines and publishes *USP DI*; Rockville, MD

- *U.S. Public Health Service*

  Offers a variety of experiences related to the provision of public healthcare; optional U.S. Public Health Service sites include the Bureau of Prisons (Washington, DC), the Food and Drug Administration (Rockville, MD), Indian Health Services (numerous locations around the U.S.), and the National Institutes of Health (Bethesda, MD)

Teach Students to Provide Pharmaceutical Care/Disease Management

During introductory practice experiences, preceptors teach pharmacy students the fundamentals of pharmacy practice. In advanced experiential rotations, preceptors continue to educate pharmacy trainees in providing patient-centered and evidence-based pharmaceutical care, which involves the following:

- Evaluating and recommending optimal medication regimens for individual patients (e.g., therapeutic selections)
- Assessing adverse reactions or drug interactions
- Identifying and evaluating clinical signs and symptoms (e.g., interview patients for a review of relevant organ systems and perform pertinent physical examinations)
- Ordering and interpreting laboratory tests in relation to medication therapy
- Assessing medication compliance for disease management and adhering to evidence-based clinical guidelines
- Establishing and evaluating therapeutic goals and outcomes (e.g., short-term treatment from an infectious cause)
- Discussing the cost of medications with other healthcare professionals and the patient prior to selection of therapy

- Monitoring medication therapy (e.g., drug concentration and organ function tests) for assessment of efficacy and toxicity
- Determine the impact of medication therapy on the patient's quality of life
- Documenting the clinical encounter (e.g., SOAP note or consultation chart note)
- Billing for pharmaceutical care services

APPEs are based on patient interaction and focused on further development of problem-solving skills. At the start of a rotation, it may be helpful to give students a pretest that includes patient case studies with medication-specific problems. The students' answers can help you assess their knowledge base and therapeutic understanding, and allow you to design educational activities for students accordingly. During the rotation, you can have student discussions by assigning readings pertinent to the specialty area of practice with questions for the student to address regarding medication-specific problems. You may also ask students to draft chart notes based on additional patient case studies and to bill for appropriate CPT codes, or to analyze their own medication prescribing recommendations and perform quality improvement using a systematic method for their own continuing professional development. Toward the end of the rotation, you could give the students a post-test to measure the progress they have made.

• Preceptor Pearls •

Pretests and post-test can be invaluable ways to assess your students' knowledge, skills, and progress.

Encourage Students to Become Independent Practitioners

The preceptor's aim during an advanced experiential rotation is to teach students how to develop independent clinical judgment while working as members of the healthcare team. This can be accomplished by directly observing a student's interventions or interactions, or through gathering feedback about student performance from other healthcare team members. The ideal preceptor-student training scenario is to have direct observation of the student by the preceptor. This enables you to have a clear perspective of the student's clinical performance, and allows you to provide specific feedback immediately to the student. It is this type of quality, timely supervision, and feedback from preceptors that improves student clinical competence, not the number of patients seen by a student.[5]

The preceptor can assist the student in applying a concept taught from their didactic education to the actual patient (e.g., see one, do one, teach one) by allowing the student the freedom to exercise his or her judgment skills. For example, students should have the opportunity to solve difficult problems on their own (e.g., how to renally adjust tobramycin therapy), and then they should discuss with you the best approach and solution to the problem. Students who lack self-confidence and always rely on others to find therapeutic answers will especially need guidance. Assign them tasks with increasing difficulty and give them positive feedback. Conversely, students who are overly confident and ignore supervision may need a reminder to check in with the preceptor and make reports to other team members. It is important for to involve students in evaluating their own learning in order to develop their skills of critical reflection for continued professional development.[6]

Teach Students to Organize Daily Activities and Manage Time Wisely

As students move from didactic to experiential learning and from introductory to advanced experiential rotations, they need to learn to manage their time wisely in order to accomplish an increasing number of tasks. During advanced rotations, they will need to review more charts, check more prescriptions, evaluate more patients, and document more chart notes—all without compromising the quality of their pharmacy skills. Make suggestions to students for maintaining quality job performance based on you own experience and help them by setting both quantitative and qualitative goals as the rotation progresses. Whatever pharmacy position a student may choose, the student needs to understand that efficient organization of daily activities and wise time management are essential to a successful career.

Influence Students to Develop a Healthy Professional Attitude

Preceptors can influence students to develop a healthy professional attitude by being enthusiastic about their work and by demonstrating a strong work ethic. As students are expected to perform a greater number of tasks during their advanced experiential training, they may face greater challenges and stress. As they attempt to further develop their professional skills and stretch their capabilities, students may become increasingly frustrated or overwhelmed. When this happens, do not lower the educational standards of the clinical training simply to alleviate student anxiety, but rather explain to students the ways in which you personally cope with stress and frustration. Healthcare professionals and model preceptors often use humor as a release for their stress and frustration.

Another point that may help relieve the frustration of struggling students is to inform these students that the most common reasons for disciplinary action from medical boards after graduation are irresponsibility, diminished capacity for self-improvement (including a poor attitude), and poor initiative as manifested by a lack of motivation or enthusiasm.[7] So, if students are responsible and motivated to help patients, they should feel somewhat reassured about their liability in their future pharmacy practice.

Empathy for patients is a professional attribute that pharmacy students can further cultivate through advanced experiential education. As students have more direct interactions with patients and their family members, students may feel more emotionally connected to them. Preceptors can help students develop professional attitudes that include having empathy and establishing healthy professional relationships with patients without becoming too emotionally involved.

Share with Students the Satisfaction of Professional Growth and Scholarly Development

Specialty education, a form of advanced experiential rotations, focuses on particular areas of expertise, allowing for concentration in both clinical learning and scholarly development. Give students opportunities to help you with a research project, whether it is a health outcomes study, a quality-control study, a translational research project, a pharmacokinetics study, or a controlled clinical trial. With instruction, students will learn the necessary steps in conducting a research study (e.g., development of research protocols, tools, and instruments; methods of data collection; choice of statistical analyses) or submitting a manuscript for publication in a peer-reviewed journal. Students can also be especially helpful in completing the background literature search, data retrieval, and analysis of the information to formulate a research hypothesis. They will also benefit from learning about the obstacles that had to be overcome in a research study and will gain satisfaction in knowing that research results can improve patient care. Another motivating factor for students is to be able to assist in the presentation of a research project at a local, state, or national pharmacy or medical meeting. These events are great opportunities for personal and professional growth. When students observe the enthusiasm that preceptors have for developing scholarly activities and gain some hands-on experience in research projects and presentations, they will be inspired to develop their own scholarly agenda.

Teach Students to Teach Others

Teaching students how to teach others is an important component of advanced experiential education. Initially, you should ascertain if the student has had prior teaching opportunities and encourage him or her to reflect on what went well and what areas needed improvement. Then, you can use several methods to hone the teaching skills of your students. First, allow students to watch you teach. Second, explain the teaching techniques you use and describe how you prepare to teach a class or educate a patient. Third, give students opportunities to teach through in-service presentations, patient education encounters, and in introductory rotations with other students. Lastly, students should interact with students from other colleges of pharmacy to teach each other through patient care rounds, topic discussions and patient presentations. Giving students feedback after their presentations will also help them improve their teaching and presentation styles.

Interpersonal Skills

How a pharmacist interacts with other professionals in a multidisciplinary healthcare setting can affect his or her professional future. Teamwork is essential in such a setting, and preceptors should help students develop the personable, working style that makes teamwork possible. Preceptors should be a positive role model, using effective listening, nonverbal, questioning, and narrative skills to communicate with patients, families, and other healthcare professionals about medication management. Preceptors should also demonstrate sensitivity by recognizing the influence of a patient's culture, age, gender, and disability on his or her health beliefs as it relates to pharmacotherapy. How well preceptors interact with others in these situations can have far-reaching effects on the future professional performance of their students. For this reason, always role model appropriate interpersonal skills. During experiential rotations, observe and provide feedback to students regarding their interpersonal interactions with other pharmacy staff, other healthcare professionals, and patients.

• Preceptor Pearls •

Helping students develop their interpersonal skills involves role modeling, observation, and feedback.

Unfortunately, sometimes teamwork-related processes can be challenging for both preceptors and students. Preceptors and students may struggle to work effectively with others or even with each other, especially if personalities clash. If this occurs, you must have the personal confidence, emotional vulnerability, and integrity to be honest and human with yourself, and to explore the possibility that you may have contributed to the problem. Having the ability to overcome these challenges is important to the professional development of both students and preceptors.

Advanced Experiential Sites

The selection of advanced experiential sites should emphasize and reflect the philosophy of the pharmacy school program. This creates consistent pharmacy ideals for students as they transfer from their didactic teaching to their APPE training. This strategy can help students develop their skills in advanced practice areas, empowering students to contribute effectively in a dynamic healthcare system. Through these experiential rotations, students should progress from student interns to professional pharmacists with the associated responsibility of accountability.

• Preceptor Pearls •

Advanced experiential rotations provide the opportunity for students to develop from interns to professional pharmacists.

Most colleges and schools of pharmacy have specific requirements for the number and types of rotations a student has to complete during the final year of training. The main difference among practice experiences is usually whether there is a direct patient care component to the rotation (see Box 6.2 for the list of examples of advanced experiential rotations). Rotations that require the student to provide distributive services (dispensing prescriptions, performing prospective drug use reviews, compounding sterile parenterals, etc.) are required rotations for most programs. Additionally, many boards of pharmacy require the intern to be under the direct supervision of the preceptor when performing these duties. Most traditional community and institutional pharmacy rotations fall under this category. Depending on the program requirements and the student's experience prior to entering the final year, a student may have the option of "placing out" of one or both of these rotation experiences by successfully passing a qualifying examination. This provides the student with an opportunity to pursue other areas of interest while meeting the requirements of the program.

Today's Pharm.D. curricula require the student to complete several clinical rotations in both the acute care/inpatient and ambulatory care environment. The student will usually complete some form of an internal medicine rotation that will involve exposure to several common disease states (e.g., hypertension, hyperlipidemia, diabetes, asthma, coronary artery disease, etc.). The student may need to complete this type of rotation in an inpatient and ambulatory area, depending on the program requirements. In addition, other clinical specialties routinely qualify as clinical rotation experiences including, but not limited to, the following: pediatrics, psychiatry, oncology, infectious diseases, critical care, and nutrition support.

Elective rotations may or may not have a direct patient care component. Some programs allow rotations that would count as a required rotation to also qualify as an elective rotation. A student may request to have a direct patient care component for all rotations depending on his or her career goals. Other students may have interest in other aspects of pharmacy practice. An elective rotation allows a student to pursue his or her interests while meeting the requirements of the degree program. State boards of pharmacy usually do not count these types of rotations as earned intern hours even though the academic program may require this type of rotation. Examples of elective rotations include drug and poison information (although some programs consider this to be a direct patient care rotation if the information provided by the student will be used to make a clinical decision for a patient in the institution), pharmaceutical sales and education, association management, legislative and regulatory practice, academic teaching, as well as basic science research.

There are several types of competitive rotation experiences that students may complete as part of their experiential training. Many pharmaceutical companies offer competitive internships that provide degree credits and experience for students with an interest in the pharmaceutical industry. Many of the national and state pharmaceutical organizations offer internships in association management and/or elective rotations. ASHP, APhA, and NACDS currently offer student rotations as well as executive residencies. The federal government and armed services have competitive rotations for students with the FDA, the Veteran's Administration, and the Indian Health Service.

Effective Methods, Styles, and Strategies of Teaching and Learning

Teaching can be rewarding, especially if you feel that you are able to pass on substantive skills and knowledge to the student. Effective teaching inspires the curiosity of students and helps improve problem solving skills that they can use in all healthcare settings. The most important goal of a preceptor is to inspire students to consistently learn by questioning their environments and assessing their personal approach to patient care.

Types of Learners

There are three types of learners: visual, auditory, and kinesthetic. Knowing the learning style your student prefers will help facilitate your teaching and the student's learning process. Most students learn from a mixture of styles but tend to process information with predominantly one style. Adjusting your teaching methods to the topic you are discussing and encompassing multiple teaching formats including reading, writing, charts, diagrams, and interactive discussions will help create the ideal learning environment for your students (Table 6.1).

Visual learners tend to learn from written words, graphs, charts, text books, and spatial arrangements. You should teach to this type of learner by giving reading assignments and having the student use visual aids like graphs, pictures, and written responses to questions.

Auditory learners acquire new information from listening. Teaching exercises that work well for this type of student include having discussions on topics and having students repeat back what they have learned. Use presentations like journal club and case presentations as major learning activities.

Kinesthetic learners process information by doing activities instead of just listening or reading. They prefer a hands-on approach and do well when they participate in rounds communicating with

Table 6.1 • *How to Present Information to Different Types of Students*	
Type of Learner	Ways to Present Information
Visual: "Write It"	• Provide written materials and exercises • Write key words on board or flip chart • Ask student to write a response • Use visuals or graphics • Ask student to be recorder in a group • Involve student through visual/spatial sense
Auditory: "Say It"	• State the information • Ask audience to describe specific info • Provide discussion periods • Encourage questions • Foster small group participation • Utilize audiovisuals and other audio methods
Kinesthetic: "Demonstrate It"	• Demonstrate how a principle works • Ask student to practice the technique • Encourage underlining and highlighting key words • Provide real-life simulations • Offer hands-on activities • Involve student physically

Adapted with permission from Karen Hamilton.[8]

physicians and other healthcare providers. One of the activities they might benefit from is shadowing other disciplines that encourage them to do more hands-on patient care activities. They also do well with interactive discussions from which they can then apply the knowledge learned to a patient situation.

• Preceptor Pearls •

Knowing the learning style your student prefers will help facilitate your teaching and the student's learning process.

Logic-Based Method to Teaching

One of the most effective methods of teaching is a logic-based system. This method is especially conducive for the practice of medicine in which statistics and evidence-based medicine are integral. There are three components to this problem solving technique: identifying the problem, identifying why the problem occurred, and lastly, identifying solutions to the problem.

The first step in building problem solving skills in students is to help them identify problems that impact the care of the patient (Box 6.5). Prepare activities and exercises that help students detect issues they need to address. Using real patient scenarios to find active problems will make the experience more meaningful. An example of a problem solving activity with a student in a retail/ community setting is to have the student who is filling prescriptions go over the patient's other medications for drug interactions, duplications, and to make sure that the patient is on appropriate medications for his or her disease states. For example, if the patient has metformin and insulin on the medication profile but not aspirin, the student can talk with the patient, ask appropriate questions, and initiate an intervention if appropriate.

Box 6.5 • Sample Activities to Help Identify Problems in Common Practice Settings

Community/Ambulatory/Hospital setting:

1. Review medication profile

2. Manage disease states

3. Assess patient compliance

4. Assess patient comprehension

The second step in problem solving is developing a method that helps the student assess underlying causes for the problem that will help in understanding the full scope. Each health-related problem has many compounding aspects, and exposing the student to these aspects gives them a comprehensive and in-depth view of the patient's condition. A tool that looks at the whole patient and the interconnecting play between medications, patient medical and social history, physical exam, and laboratories, is the Problem Solving Triad (Figure 6.1), which can apply to any setting for dissecting a medical problem.

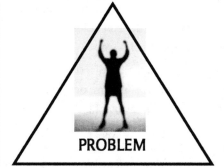

Medications:
Complete list of medications, including OTC/herbals

History/Physical Exam:
BP, HR, RR Temperature
Pain
Blood sugars
Bowel movements
Sleeping/eating
Social and medical history

PROBLEM

Labs:
Chemistry
CBC
Lipid panel
Liver panel
Cultures

Figure 6.1. The problem solving triad.

Understanding each of the three aspects of the Problem Solving Triad allows us to approach the patient and their management from a whole perspective. Fully assessing labs and vital signs is important to determine the impact of the therapeutic regimen on the patient's underlying health condition. An exercise demonstrating the Problem Solving Triad in each practice setting is provided below using the patient complaint of diarrhea.

Scenario for community setting. Problem: Diarrhea

1. History/physical exam: Patient reports loose bowel movements for 5 days; decreased blood pressure and increased heart rate when checked at counter; no change in PO intake.

2. Labs: No current labs available, but patient reports that last week she had an elevated white blood count. She states that she is currently being treated for a urinary tract infection.

3. Medications: From the patient's filled prescription record, she is on Bactrim DS, metformin, lisinopril, atorvastatin, aspirin, and metoprolol.

Same scenario for clinic/hospital setting. Problem: Diarrhea

1. History/physical exam: Past medical history of diabetes, hypertension, coronary artery disease, and current urinary tract infection; loose bowel movement for 5 days; decreased blood pressure and increased heart rate since yesterday; fluid intake is 1.5 L/day

2. Labs: hypomagnesaemia; hypokalemia; increased BUN/ serum creatinine ratio >20; leukocytosis but trending down

3. Medications: Bactrim DS, metformin, lisinopril, atorvastatin, aspirin, and metoprolol

The patient complaint of diarrhea can be further examined with the Problem Solving Triad. The health complications of the diarrhea can be used to help us elucidate the possible cause. The loss of fluids from the diarrhea has affected the patient's blood pressure and heart rate. The patient has not increased his or her food or water intake to compensate for the losses, resulting in dehydration, which is reflected in the lab values (increased BUN/ SCr, decreased potassium and magnesium). By looking at the medications, students can ascertain potential causes of the diarrhea (e.g., antibiotics or metformin). By examining the history, students can rule out potential causes such as gastroenteritis, or manifestations of disease states such as Crohn's disease or diverticulitis.

Once students have a list of potential causes of diarrhea, they can decide the most likely etiology based on the patient's subjective and objective information. Even in a community setting where only limited physical exam and lab information are available, the student can learn to solve complex health problems using the right tools and strategies. The Problem Solving Triad is useful in incorporating medications with all other health parameters. This tool allows pharmacy students to go beyond just examining the patient medication list, assessing each patient health issue from a comprehensive perspective. This will allow students to effectively solve patient problems and thus make a significant impact on patient care.

• Preceptor Pearls •

Use the Problem Solving Triad as a systematic method for problem solving that you can apply to many different situations.

The last step in problem solving is developing solutions that are feasible for the patient and healthcare provider. It is important to remember that many patient problems are complex and having only one solution to the problem may leave other more viable and appropriate solutions undiscovered. Prepare activities for students that involve coming up with multiple solutions to a problem. This prompts students to think about confounders such as drug allergies, disease state contraindications, drug interactions, cost prohibitions, insurance formulary restrictions, and compliance issues. Challenging the student to identify at least three solutions to most problems allows the student to move past the most easily identifiable solution and to learn how to come up with novel potential solutions. In the case of the patient with diarrhea, suppose the cause is the antibiotics. Three possible solutions are (1) since there are only a few days left to complete treatment, consider staying on Bacrtim DS but increase hydration and add antidiarrheal; (2) contact physician and consider change of antibiotics; and (3) keep same antibiotic, add lactobacillus treatment, increase hydration, and PRN antidiarrheal. Depending on the patient's severity of diarrhea and the patient's economic and social conditions, any number of these interventions may be appropriate. The student should assess each intervention in the context of the patient's entire clinical and social picture, and then work with the patient and the physician to determine the best intervention.

Tools for Teaching and Learning

New Technologies

It is vital to familiarize our students with new technologies and computer-based processes since they are now an integral part of healthcare practice. Students must learn how to incorporate technologies such as handheld drug information devices and Internet resources, which are frequently used by healthcare professionals for learning and gathering data. In many ways, these technologies offer a more efficient means of obtaining drug and medical information because healthcare professionals can obtain information rapidly and the resources are more portable then print resources such as the *Drug Information Handbook*. Some pharmacy schools are now requiring students to purchase a personal digital assistant (PDA), and most schools strongly promote computer use in order to familiarize students with accessing electronic drug and medical information. Even though the expanding influence of the Internet and handheld devices on healthcare practice is inevitable, preceptors must teach students not only how to use such information, but also how to use more traditional information resources, because many pharmacy practice sites do not have access to all desired information electronically.

Use of Nonpharmacy Personnel

One of the biggest lessons for students to learn is the importance of their contributions to the care of the patient. Understanding where pharmacy fits in the whole spectrum of care will make them not only appreciate their role but also enhance their perception of other ways pharmacists can contribute to healthcare. Students who have exposure to and/or have shadowed nonpharmacy personnel such as physicians, respiratory technicians, nurses, case managers, speech and physical therapists, and dietitians, find themselves feeling more like part of the patient care team. Pharmacists impact other disciplines in many ways. Some examples include the schedules we set for dose administration by nursing and respiratory technicians, and the types of medications we choose that can aid or hinder the care provided by therapists or dietitians. Teaching students about other healthcare professionals' roles will help students communicate with them, and will advance students' abilities to optimize pharmacotherapy regimens for both the patient and for other healthcare professionals providing care.

The greatest reward for the preceptor is to know that our teaching style and methods have provided our students with a positive experience and have inspired them to excel in their future pharmacy careers.

Student Evaluation

In their book, *The One Minute Manager*, Blanchard and Johnson offer a simple approach to providing formative feedback: the One Minute Praising and the One Minute Reprimand (Table 6.2).[9] Their method can be easily adapted to the preceptor-student environment. Initiate a one-minute praise when you catch students performing a desired behavior. Praise student behavior as soon as possible, being very specific about what was done right. Emphasize how the behavior positively impacts patient care or others in the practice setting. Follow with a short pause to let students savor the moment. Then, encourage students to continue this positive behavior.

Table 6.2 • *The One Minute Praising and Reprimand*	
The One Minute Praising	The One Minute Reprimand
Praise the behavior	*Reprimand the behavior*
Do it soon	*Do it soon, but wait until you are calm and in private*
Be specific about what the person did right	*Be specific about what the person did wrong*
Tell the person how you feel	*Tell the person how you feel*
Pause to let the person "feel" how good you feel	*Pause to let the person "feel" how you feel*
Encourage more of the same	*Encourage improvement*

Unfortunately, it is also a preceptor's responsibility to identify student weaknesses so that students can correct them. The One Minute Reprimand offers an effective way for you to carry out this important responsibility. You should initiate the reprimand as soon as possible after identifying the behavior. However, wait until you are calm and seek a private place to talk with the student. Be very specific about what the student did wrong. Again, it is important to let the student know how his or her behavior impacts patient care or others in the practice site. Although it may be uncomfortable, pause to let the student know how you feel is important. After this pause, assure the student that you are there to help him or her succeed. You may wish to point out that it is the student's behavior that is the focus of the reprimand, not the student personally. Finally, do not dwell on the reprimand. When it is over, it is over.

Summative Evaluation

Summative evaluation assesses competency achievement. It is often the primary determination of whether or not students successfully complete a given practice experience. For this reason, preceptors must be as objective as possible and perform these evaluations with great care and concern. Never take lightly your responsibility to assess student competency. Although it is not easy to fail students, you must if a student does not achieve the competencies, and your obligation to patients, the profession, and the students demand it.

• Preceptor Pearls •

Although a summative evaluation may determine the final decision of whether to fail a student or not, feedback throughout the rotation should ensure that no one is surprised by the outcome.

Timing of Summative Evaluation

Timing of summative evaluation is important and depends on the nature and length of the practice experience as well as the method of evaluation used. In all cases, summative evaluation should be based on specific objectives or competencies established for the practice experience. Discuss these objectives with students at the beginning of the practice experience. Then, tell students when and how you will evaluate them on these competencies. You should conduct at least some method of summative evaluation at the midpoint of the rotation. Students need to know how they are progressing. Make a plan to correct weaknesses you identify. Do not wait until the end of a practice experience to let students know they are doing poorly. Surprises at the end of the practice experience are never productive for students or preceptors.

Conduct a final summative evaluation at the end of the practice experience. This evaluation should reflect the students' actual ability to achieve the competencies established for the rotation. Resist the temptation to reward or grade students based on improvement. Remember, you are evaluating the students' ability to demonstrate competency in performing specific behaviors, not their ability to show improvement or display effort.

Methods of Summative Evaluation

Summative evaluation may follow a number of different methods. The method you choose will depend on the nature of the practice experience and the frequency of evaluation. Often, a combination of methods may be used to provide a broader and more accurate assessment of student abilities.

Examination (written, oral, and practical). In the classroom, students are tested primarily through written examination. This method may also be used in the clinical setting. Individual preceptors may prepare and administer written exams, or in many cases, the college of pharmacy may do so. Use written exams to test knowledge of pharmaceutical calculations, pharmacy laws and regulations, and drug-specific information. Written exams may also test student ability to use reference materials to answer specific questions or to provide drug information. Written exams are often part of the final summative evaluation process used to determine a student's grade for the practice experience.

Oral examinations may be a more useful method of summative evaluation in the clinical setting. Use oral examinations to test not only specific drug knowledge, but also students' decision-making and problem-solving abilities. Ask probing questions to ensure students have a thorough understanding of the situation discussed. Alter scenarios or add information to test their ability to reformulate decisions. An oral examination may be part of the final summative evaluation process, but you can also use it more informally throughout the practice experience to assess and guide student learning.

Practical examinations allow students to demonstrate their ability in performing very specific, physical behaviors. Use this method to test skills such as sterile and nonsterile compounding, patient counseling, and professional interactions with other healthcare providers. Establish specific criteria for each behavior or skill and grade according to these criteria. Like oral examinations, this method can be part of the final summative evaluation process or occur throughout the practice experience to assess and guide student learning.

Evaluation instruments. An evaluation instrument is perhaps the most common method of summative evaluation for assessment of student competency in the pharmacy practice setting. The college of pharmacy usually provides such instruments, which use a numeric, alphabetic, or Likert scale. The school may ask preceptors to evaluate students' application of knowledge, technical skills, and attitudes and personal attributes. By nature, this type of instrument is prone to subjectivity and bias. In addition, the school may ask you to evaluate behaviors that occurred several weeks prior to the time of evaluation. You must do all you can to make the evaluation process objective and reflective of student behaviors as they actually occurred. A five-step approach to completing student evaluations has been suggested[10]:

1. **Observe the students.** Observe students performing the behaviors to be evaluated at least several times over the evaluation period. Ask others who interact with the students to observe student behavior. Do they observe the same things you do?

2. **Record observations.** Make a record of the behaviors you observe. Do this soon after you observe the behavior. Use index cards or a PDA to make recording of behaviors easy. Abbreviate and use codes, but remember to be specific. Ask others who interact with the students to record student behaviors. At this point, do not evaluate behaviors—just record them.

3. **Retrieve recorded observations.** Collect the records of your observations and the observations of others. Sort and organize them as they relate to the competencies to be evaluated. Do this weekly to identify behaviors that you have not yet observed or need more observation. Use what you learn to guide student learning experiences over the remainder of the rotation.

4. **Analyze retrieved observations.** Look for patterns of performance. Do students consistently perform or fail to perform a specific behavior as required? Do students perform the behavior on their own or do they need assistance and prompting from preceptors or others? Do the recorded behaviors reflect students' typical performance?

5. **Evaluate the students.** Use what you learn from step 4 to complete the evaluation instrument. Develop a strategy that works for the type of scale you used. For example, if you used a numeric scale, start with the highest ranking and consider whether students

have obtained this level of competence. If not, move to the next lower ranking. Continue until you have selected the ranking that best reflects student behavior. If space is provided for comment, describe specific behaviors that support your rating.

No matter what type of rating scale you use, evaluation instruments are subject to error and bias. Familiarity with the types of errors that can occur will help you to avoid them when you evaluate students (Box 6.6).

Box 6.6 • Errors in Evaluation

- Error of harshness and leniency. A preceptor who assigns a higher rating to a student he or she likes or knows well has committed an error of leniency. In some cases, a preceptor may overcompensate for his or her personal feelings toward a student by assigning that student a lower rating.

- Central tendency. This error occurs when a preceptor avoids giving a student extreme ratings, instead assigning the student ratings in the middle of the rating scale. A preceptor who has little firsthand knowledge of a student's performance in a given competency error may be more likely to commit this error.

- Halo effect. The halo effect occurs when a preceptor evaluates a competency based on a student's performance in another area. For example, a preceptor may negatively evaluate a student's ability to maintain professional and ethical standards because of the student's poor dress or appearance.

- Logical error. This error occurs when a preceptor gives similar ratings for competencies that seem related to one another. For example, a preceptor may give a student a high rating in nonsterile compounding because the student received a high rating for sterile compounding. Again, this error may occur more often in cases where a preceptor has little firsthand knowledge of a student's ability in a given competency area.

- Proximity error. Preceptors who assign similar ratings to competencies that are located next to each other on the evaluation instrument have committed a proximity error.

- Contrast error. A contrast error occurs when a preceptor rates a student negatively on a competency that the preceptor does extremely well. For example, the preceptor has an exceptional ability to communicate with patients and rates the student negatively on this competency because the student could not perform this function as well as the preceptor.

- Grading on improvement. This error occurs when a preceptor assigns a rating based on a student's effort or improvement rather than on the student's actual ability to perform the task to the level required.

• Preceptor Pearls •

Ensure you evaluate your student objectively, avoiding error and bias.

After you have completed the evaluation instrument, you should share it with the student. Find a quiet, private place to talk with the student. Review your ratings and comments with the student. Be specific. Provide examples from the observations you recorded that support your ratings. Point out behaviors the student does well in addition to behaviors the student needs to improve. Involve the student in formulating a plan to improve areas of weakness. If necessary, re-evaluate areas of weakness on a weekly basis to ensure improvement as planned.

Secrets of Success

Providing student feedback and evaluation does not have to be a frustrating and overwhelming task. Techniques such as the One Minute Praising and Reprimand allow you to provide students with ongoing feedback in a quick and effective manner. At the beginning of the practice experience, tell students what summative evaluation methods you will use and how you will determine their grade. Remember that the process of summative evaluation does not begin at the midpoint or end of the practice experience. Observe and record student behaviors throughout the entire practice experience. Retrieve and analyze these behaviors in order to complete the evaluation instrument. When appropriate, use written, oral, and practical examinations to aid in student evaluation. An organized, behavior-focused approach to student evaluation encourages open preceptor-student communication and ensures a less frustrating and fearful experience for both.

Potential Precepting Challenges

When you decide to take a student on an experiential rotation, you expect that the student will work very hard and have an excellent learning experience. Unfortunately, sometimes this does not occur. When faced with a difficult student, many times you may be unsure what to do to handle the student or situation. In addition, it is not uncommon to blame the student and/or yourself for the problems that are occurring. The dangers associated with this type of scenario are that the student may have a negative experience and fail the rotation and you may decide to stop teaching students.

There are many reasons why a student may have difficulty during a rotation. When there are problems, the origin of the difficulty usually falls into one or more of the following areas:

- Attitude and motivation
- Attention to the academic program
- Comprehension

Attitudinal Issues

A student who begins a rotation with a poor attitude will present many challenges for the preceptor. For some students, a bad attitude may not have caused problems during the didactic portion of their training. Performing below expectations and being informed that his or her attitude is poor may come as a surprise to some of them. The student with this type of attitude frequently disregards instructions from the preceptor (arrives late, does the minimal amount of work, appears lazy) and may become defensive when confronted about his or her behavior. This student has survived for years with this type of attitude and may feel personally attacked by the preceptor. Lack of motivation is evident in everything he or she does (or does not do). The preceptor may have to be repetitive regarding instructions and usually ends up very frustrated.

Even though this type of student may deserve to fail based on attitude, unfortunately his or her performance may not meet the criteria for failure as outlined by the training program. The student who does the least amount of work possible may still meet the minimal requirements of the rotation and be eligible for a passing grade. This presents a difficult ethical issue for the preceptor and program (e.g. the student meets the minimal requirements for passing; however, he or she demonstrates a very unprofessional attitude).

Assessment of behavior and conduct are routine criteria for most programs. The examples listed in the above case (reporting late, not completing assignments, etc.) could be classified as "unprofessional conduct" and be grounds for failure of a rotation. Failing a student is always difficult because you want to see the student succeed and as you may feel that you have done something wrong. It is essential to review professional expectations with the students prior to starting rotations (hopefully these are emphasized from the moment they start the pharmacy program). Penalties for unprofessional conduct should be specified in the course and/or rotation syllabus. This information should be shared with the student and their preceptors. The following information is an example of this information; it is included in the course syllabus for all rotations at the University of Texas at Austin College of Pharmacy[11]:

> Student-intern professional conduct. Student-interns must also abide by all laws and regulations pertaining to a pharmacist-intern as defined by the Texas Pharmacy Act and Rules. Violation of these laws and regulations may jeopardize the intern's privilege to become a registered pharmacist in Texas and may also result in failure of the course and dismissal from the College and/or the University.

> **Special Note:** Students will be removed from a rotation for conduct deemed unprofessional by the preceptor and/or Student Affairs Office, OR if the student's actions endanger patient health/welfare. Removal from a rotation for either of these two reasons will result in possible failure of the rotation.

It is critical to document specific instances of unprofessional behavior and communicate this information with the college/school administration. Preceptors should never feel as if they are punished when these situations occur. Failing a rotation is an academic decision and the responsibility rests with the college/school.

Attention to the Academic Program

Today's student is very different from students 20 years ago. Many students have already been through the academic process, having completed bachelor's and master's degrees prior to entering the pharmacy program. Some students have already spent a significant amount of time in the workforce and are back in college to facilitate a career change. This student may not be as concerned with earning the highest grades in the class as he or she has other external pressures outside of his or her studies. Today's student is often married with children and/or other dependents to support. This student may be more concerned with passing courses and rotations than with trying to excel. In essence, this student excels in simply making it through the program because of the number of responsibilities that he or she has to juggle. It is easy to see how the attention of this type of student can be pulled in multiple directions and away from the academic program.

Comprehension

A surprising and troubling issue for preceptors is encountering the student who performs poorly in the final year of the program. There are generally two types of students who fit into this category: the 4.0 student and the 2.0 student. The 4.0 student may have done well in didactic courses yet cannot apply that knowledge in a real patient-care situation. These students may be labeled "book smart"— knowing lots of information but lacking practical application skills. Students who fall into this category may have been able to memorize large amounts of information and to regurgitate these facts on exams. Integrating this information and applying it to patients who do not present as a typical "textbook" case can bewilder the student. This student is stunned to learn that his or her performance is lacking and he or she may be in danger of not passing the rotation.

The 2.0 student may have worked very hard during the didactic courses yet never performed well on exams. His or her comprehension of information may be limited; however, he or she has been able to score well enough to progress through the program. This is the student who may be "exposed" or "found out" during the experiential rotations. For some, failure to perform satisfactorily on rotations does not come as a surprise and actually may be a relief. For others, they will need to take on the impossible task of learning four years of pharmacy curricula in a 4- to 6-week rotation. This student will end up facing one failure after another and, depending on the circumstances and requirements of the program, may be subject to dismissal in the final year of training.

Practice Setting Issues

For any of the students described above, a busy practice environment can be a prescription for failure. All of these students may be immediately overwhelmed with the pace and expectations of their preceptor and the rotation. Intervention by the preceptor and/or program can cause the student to become frustrated and disengaged. These situations may be compounded if the student is on a rotation with any classmates. Even the best preceptor can fall into the trap of comparing students that are from the same program, which only makes the situation more difficult for the student who is consistently performing below expectations. In addition, the student who is performing poorly may be intimidated by how well his or her peers are doing and reluctant to ask for assistance from anyone.

Strategies for Dealing with Difficult Students and Situations

The first consideration when facing difficult students or situations is to determine what may be causing the student to perform poorly. Once you identify the underlying etiology, you can decide what type of intervention is necessary. In all cases, you should immediately notify the program's coordinator at the academic institution that the student is having problems. The program coordinator is in the best position to advise you on how to handle the situation. In most cases, you will need to document the areas in which the student is not performing satisfactorily in the student's assessment or evaluation form. A comprehensive review and understanding of what the academic program requires and its assessment tool is critical.

Consider the following when dealing with difficult students:

- Did I clearly outline the objectives and expectations for the rotation?
- Does the student have direct patient care responsibilities and can the student continue with the rotation without compromising patient care?

- Is this the first exposure the student has had to this type of practice environment?

- Where is the student in the sequence of rotations (i.e., first versus last rotation)?

- Have I reviewed the student's performance on prior rotations and/or detected any prior problems and/or issues?

- Have I been available to provide feedback as the student encounters new and unfamiliar situations?

- Have I been approachable or does the student appear to be afraid to ask questions?

- Do I frequently provide feedback and make time to meet with the student to review his or her progress?

- Have other members of the pharmacy staff been supportive and helpful to the student?

Once you have identified the problem, you can institute necessary measures to deal with the issue. As previously discussed, the student may not be aware of his or her failure to meet performance expectations. In many cases, the student will need to deal with this emotional issue before making any progress toward resolving the difficulty and hopefully moving forward with the training. If appropriate, schedule a meeting with the student to discuss the issues in as nonthreatening of an environment as possible. Do this as early as feasible to address student difficulties and, when possible, provide time for improvement. This meeting should occur in private unless the problem warrants having a witness or a member of the academic training program present. Confronting a difficult student or one who is failing is not easy for any preceptor. Delaying the discussion with the student will only feed the problem and not solve it. Additionally, it is unfair to the student to expect improvement on an issue that he or she may not be aware is occurring.

Consider the following when meeting with difficult students:

- Agree on a time with the student to conduct a private meeting. Let the student know that the meeting is to discuss a specific issue and not a routine meeting to assess progress.

- Let the student know your perception of the problem at the beginning of the meeting. Try to be objective and clear of what the nature of the problem is and provide examples.

- Let the student know at the beginning the seriousness of the problem. Is the issue something that may cause harm to a patient, the department, and other staff? What are the implications for the student (e.g., failure of the rotation)?

- Give the student an opportunity to digest the news and present his or her perception of the issue. Is there a factor of which the preceptor is unaware that is preventing the student from performing in a satisfactory manner?

- Do not interrupt and/or get defensive when the student is talking. This may be the first time the student is hearing that there is a problem and will need time to digest this information. It is natural for the student to become defensive and very emotional. Allow the emotions to surface and give the student the opportunity to express them and then calm down. The student will not hear you while in a highly emotional state.

- Document your discussion and take notes, if appropriate, as the student presents his or her side of the story. This will help you focus on the problem and provide concrete information for resolution of the issue.

- Get the student's input regarding how to address the problem. Develop a plan of what the student needs to do in order to successfully complete the rotation.

- Document the plan and get the student to sign it. This is essential if further action may be required (e.g., assignment of a failing grade, dismissal from the site, etc.). Additionally, having the student sign the plan will help convey the seriousness of the issue.

- Schedule a timeframe for improvement and times to meet to monitor progress.

- Thank the student for his or her time and remind him or her that you are there to provide assistance.

The Failing Student

Sometimes students fail no matter how hard a preceptor tries to help. When confronted with a student who is having significant difficulty with a rotation, remember that preceptors do not assign failing grades; students earn them. Students fail because they are not meeting the requirements of the rotation. Having to give a student a failing grade is very difficult for a preceptor. Even if the student has shown some improvement, there are times when the student should not receive a passing grade and may need to repeat the rotation. The most important factor for the preceptor to consider is whether you want this student to provide patient care with the type of performance you have observed. If the answer is "no," you should not give the student a passing grade, and the student should not progress in the program. Preceptors have an essential role in the educational process. The preceptor is the one who has the final say regarding whether a student is ready to graduate and enter the profession. This is a huge responsibility and one that you should not take lightly. As much as a preceptor has a responsibility to educate future practitioners, the preceptor's role in preventing nonqualified individuals from entering practice is as important, if not more important.

• Preceptor Pearls •

Remember that preceptors do not assign failing grades; students earn them.

How to Develop, Implement, Coordinate, and Monitor an Introductory or Advanced Internship Program

Developing, implementing, coordinating, and monitoring an introductory or advanced pharmacy practice internship program at your practice site can be an exciting, challenging, and fulfilling experience. For preceptors who have never done this before, the director of experiential education at the pharmacy school and materials developed by the faculty can be great resources. In fact, inviting the director of experiential education to your practice site to see it and discuss the possibilities and school requirements can be a good way to begin planning your practice site. Also, networking with more seasoned preceptors is a great way to benefit from the successes and mistakes of others, get useful tips, and avoid potential pitfalls. Additionally, preceptors with a similar internship to the one you are designing may be willing to share some of the materials that they have previously developed (e.g., orientation checklist, evaluation forms, program manual).

Designing the Program Curriculum

Designing the program curriculum begins with reviewing the materials from the pharmacy school with which your practice site is affiliated. For required introductory or advanced practice experiences, the pharmacy school should have a course description and a syllabus that outlines the course goals and objectives, activities, assignments, textbooks and/or other reading materials, terminal competencies, written and/or oral exams, grading procedures, and relevant course and school policies (e.g., attendance, tardiness, absences, makeup work, dress code, conduct, confidentiality). This information may be packaged into a program manual provided by the school that also contains assignment and presentation guidelines; assessment instruments for the various activities and assignments; weekly hours and activity sheets; site and preceptor evaluation forms; a summative intern evaluation form; important dates; and contact information for the course coordinator and the director of the experiential education program.

For elective APPEs, especially advanced specialty practice rotations, the school may or may not have a program manual developed. The pharmacy school may only provide the relevant policies related to all internship programs and the required forms that must be completed for any experiential course (e.g., weekly hours and activity sheets, site and preceptor evaluation forms, summative intern evaluation form). In that case, the preceptor will need to define and develop the course goals and objectives, activities, assignments, reading materials, terminal competencies, written and/or oral exams, and grading procedures. Although this can take some time, it is worthwhile if the internship is in demand and will be offered frequently in the future.

Pharmacy schools strive for standardization and consistency in the way preceptors at various practice sites deliver the required internship experiences. Preceptors adhering to the requirements in the program manual ensure that all interns have a similar core experience. However, schools also realize that all preceptors and practice sites are different and have the opportunity to offer unique experiences to interns. Preceptors can have students participate in more activities and complete other assignments that the preceptor thinks are important learning experiences. The key is that these unique experiences must be in addition to the activities and assignments the school requires and not a replacement of them. You must maintain the core curriculum of the experiential learning clerkship but may create supplements as desired.

• Preceptor Pearls •

Use the information the school of pharmacy provides to you to create your program, but be creative in supplementing activities. You have the opportunity to make your internship unique and invaluable to both you and your student.

Pharmacy schools are usually not as concerned about the standardization and consistency of elective advanced specialty practice internships preceptors can deliver at various sites. This is mainly because these internships are elective and are offered by relatively few preceptors and practice sites. Preceptors are free to build these rotations around their personal strengths and the uniqueness of their practice sites and to tailor them to the needs and desires of the interns. However, they still need a course curriculum that is defined prior to the start of the internship so that the expectations are clear (e.g., course goals and objectives, activities, assignments, reading materials, terminal competencies, written and/or oral exams, grading procedures). Additionally, preceptors may be able to improve their elective advanced specialty practice internship by working together with preceptors of similar elective rotations and sharing and combining the ideas and materials developed by each other.

Constructing the Program Manual

Many preceptors use the program manual provided to them by the pharmacy school, which is perfectly appropriate. Some preceptors take the school's program manual and incorporate it into a more comprehensive program manual that they have customized for their rotation and practice site (a real "survival manual"). Whichever method you use, you can place all the materials into a three-ring binder that has tabs dividing the sections. Box 6.7 lists sample components that could be included in a program manual. By developing a program manual, you can use their creativity and express yourself in a way that might facilitate building a good preceptor-intern relationship and decrease the initial anxiety of the intern. This also is an opportunity to reveal your artistic side and your sense of humor as well as demonstrate your commitment, enthusiasm, and forethought toward the student and clerkship.

Box 6.7 • Sample Components for a Program Manual

- Welcome letter
- Diagram and directory of the healthcare organization
- Map and guide for the area
- Orientation checklist
- Forms that must be completed (e.g., self-assessment, hours sheet, practice site evaluation, preceptor evaluation, intern evaluation)
- Copy of state regulations related to intern duties
- Brief biographical statements about the preceptors
- List of the names of all pharmacy employees and their positions
- Brief description of the pharmacy department and the healthcare organization
- Copies of the Pledge of Professionalism, Oath of a Pharmacist, and Code of Ethics for Pharmacists
- Goals and objectives of the internship
- Competencies that must be demonstrated
- Required activities, assignments, and exams
- Copies of articles or presentations to read and discuss
- Sample assignment write-ups (e.g., research papers, formulary monographs, case studies, clinical intervention reports), problem sets, and exam questions

Box 6.7 • Sample Components for a Program Manual (cont'd)

- Example formats for organizing oral presentations (e.g., patient cases, journal articles, inservices) and patient care notes (e.g., medication and allergy histories, progress notes, consultations)
- Detailed schedule showing all the important activities and deadlines for assignments
- Cartoons and jokes
- Inspirational stories
- Art and history relevant to pharmacy
- Anything else that you want to share with the inter to show your personality, to make learning fun, and to enhance the intern's transition and experience at your practice site

Conducting an Effective Orientation Process

The orientation process is critically important since it becomes part of the intern's first impression of the preceptor and the practice site, and it can set the tone for the rest of the internship. The orientation process may begin before the intern arrives at the practice site on the first day. You should have a brief conversation with your intern prior to the rotation. Essential information to communicate to the student includes directions to the healthcare organization, parking information, arrival time, meeting place, and contact information for the preceptor in case of mishap (e.g., intern is lost, has an accident, or gets sick). Also, this is a chance for you to ask a few questions and allay any fears or misconceptions the intern has. The orientation process should resume as early as possible on the first day of the internship. A checklist can guide the orientation process and make sure nothing is left out. Box 6.8 lists sample items that could be included in an orientation checklist. If the orientation process cannot occur immediately after the intern's arrival because you become unexpectedly busy, the intern can shadow you until there is another opportunity to continue the orientation. Having interns come back later that day or the next day sends a negative message about your level of commitment. Conducting an effective orientation process can begin the development of a good preceptor-intern relationship and start off the internship on a positive note.

Box 6.8 • Sample Items for an Orientation Checklist

- Verify that intern's license/registration is current.
- Discuss background, pharmacy experience, and career goals and plans of the intern and preceptor.
- Discuss expectations of the intern and preceptor (e.g., conduct, ethics, confidentiality).
- Tour the pharmacy and point out important areas (e.g., work space, break room, phone, bathroom, references).
- Meet the preceptors and other pharmacy staff.
- Tour the rest of the practice site and meet other key people.
- Obtain name badge and clearance codes (e.g., pharmacy, library, and computer access) and complete any other processing requirements of the healthcare organization (e.g., review immunization records).

Box 6.8 • Sample Items for an Orientation Checklist (cont'd)

- Review pertinent policy and procedure of the pharmacy department and the healthcare organization (dress code, phone use, universal precautions).
- Review the internship program manual.
- Clarify the pharmacy duties and responsibilities for which the intern will be held accountable.
- Discuss the required activities and assignments and their completion dates.
- Clarify the schedules of the intern and preceptors.
- Discuss the feedback and evaluation process.
- Provide contact information for the preceptors (e.g., work phone, pager, e-mail, home phone).

Creating an Intern Practice Model and Assigning Duties and Responsibilities

Interns know when they are doing "busy work" that is not important to the operational mission of the pharmacy and that keeps them out of the way of the preceptors. Being sent off to work on these exercises of futility (e.g., constructing forms or pamphlets that will never be used by the pharmacy) can be very frustrating to them. Interns like to be engaged in meaningful work that allows them to contribute to the pharmacy, learn new things, and grow and develop as pharmacists.

One way to assure that interns are engaged in meaningful work is to create an intern practice model with designated duties and responsibilities that they will be held accountable for completing. Depending on the type of internship and practice site, these duties and responsibilities may be related to drug distribution services, clinical pharmacy services, a blend of both, or other types of services. Assigned tasks may be constant over the course of an internship, progress in levels of duties and responsibilities, or they may change as interns are rotated to different areas. In every case, it is important to explain to them why each task is important and what knowledge, skills, and terminal competencies you expect them to gain from completing it.

Potential duties and responsibilities that could be included in an intern practice model are listed in Box 6.9. When constructing a list of duties and responsibilities for an APPE, think about what you would want an entry-level pharmacist who was just employed by your healthcare organization to be able to do. Also, think about activities that would be good learning experiences for interns and at the same time would expand or improve the services offered by your pharmacy.

Box 6.9 • Potential Duties and Responsibilities for an Intern Practice Model

- Ordering drugs and stocking them on the shelves
- Taking new prescriptions and transferring prescriptions over the phone
- Preparing, labeling, and dispensing prescriptions

Box 6.9 • Potential Duties and Responsibilities for an Intern Practice Model (cont'd)

- Obtaining medication and allergy histories from patients and other healthcare professionals
- Triaging patients and assisting them with the selection of over-the-counter products
- Performing patient counseling related to medications and devices and documenting it in the medical record
- Conducting drug regimen reviews for all patients on the assigned patient care units
- Seeing patients every day on the assigned patient care units and assessing their subjective and objective responses to medication therapy, including performing therapeutic drug monitoring as needed
- Making recommendations to physicians related to drug therapy and working with them on developing the pharmacotherapy portion of the patient care plan
- Writing progress notes and/or consultation notes as appropriate
- Serving as a liaison for the pharmacy department on the assigned patient care unit
- Providing in-services to the pharmacy and nursing staff on requested or targeted topics

Involving Pharmacy Staff and Other Healthcare Professionals and Patients in Experiential Training

Many people can be involved in various aspects in the training of interns. Inclusion of people other than the primary preceptor usually depends on the type of rotation, the kind of practice site, and the desire of others to teach. Pharmacy technicians, staff pharmacists, clinical pharmacists, pharmacy managers, nurses, nurse practitioners, physician assistants, respiratory therapists, dietitians, and physicians are among those who frequently participate in pharmacy experiential training. Interns can spend some time with different healthcare professionals for exposure to certain areas or to focus on learning specific skills. For example, interns can learn first hand about issues related to medication administration techniques and devices (e.g., infusion pumps) by working with nurses. Interns can enhance their patient assessment and physical examination skills through working with physicians, nurse practitioners, and physician assistants. Interns can sharpen their patient counseling skills related to use of a nebulizer, inhaler, and peak flow meter by working with a respiratory therapist, or related to nutrition by working with a dietitian. These other healthcare professionals can provide feedback to the primary preceptor about the intern's performance and, thus, contribute to the evaluation process.

• Preceptor Pearls •

Thinking of other healthcare professionals involved in your student's training as preceptors as well will provide the student with a well-rounded experience.

Patients can also be involved in the training of interns, particularly in the evaluation process. Although patients may not be able to assess an intern's pharmacy knowledge base or technical skills, they can evaluate an intern's professionalism, communication and listening ability, and interpersonal skills. You can have patients fill out a very short and simple intern assessment form after their interaction with an intern. The form should contain no more than a handful of items to evaluate and fit on one piece of paper or an oversized index card. Patients may be very happy to play a small role in the education and training of future pharmacists. Patients also can be involved in more complex competency assessment methods, such as practical exams (objective structured clinical exams), and patients can be trained to give verbal feedback directly to the interns.

Evaluating the Effectiveness and Success of the Program

Pharmacy schools should be able to provide preceptors with evaluation summaries of their internship program and their practice site on a periodic basis (e.g., annually). How often this occurs may be dependent on how frequently students complete an internship with the preceptor at a given practice site. Schools are always concerned about maintaining student anonymity, which can be important in getting valid evaluations. Also, most schools have hundreds of preceptors and practice sites but few personnel devoted to experiential education that can compile and send out evaluation summaries. Unfortunately, you cannot improve yourself, your internship, or your practice site without valuable and timely feedback.

If you are not receiving evaluation summaries from the pharmacy school on a regular basis, you can develop your own preceptor, internship, and practice site evaluation forms. You can distribute, complete, and turn in these forms during the last day of the rotation after the interns have received their final grade. Also, you can conduct exit interviews with the interns at the end of their last day, discuss the evaluations with them, and seek additional verbal feedback. Interns usually are very willing to do this if they have been told that it is solely for continuous quality improvement purposes to improve the preceptor, the internship, and the practice site.

Besides reviewing evaluation summaries and setting goals in terms of the scores, there may be some other metrics you can track to evaluate the effectiveness and success of the internship program. These metrics will depend on the goals you and your supervisor have for the internship program. Often the primary goal of the internship program is to improve the recruitment of pharmacy residents and/or pharmacists. You can track over time the number of positions filled by graduates from the affiliated pharmacy school. A secondary goal may be to improve the job satisfaction and retention of pharmacists by making their work more intrinsically rewarding, which can be evaluated through repeated surveys. Other indirect measures of success that could be tracked include the number of requests made per year by students to complete a required or elective internship at the practice site; the number of pharmacy schools forming partnerships with the practice site; and the total number of interns trained per year. Of course, receiving invitations to speak at school-sponsored preceptor conferences and being presented with preceptor awards would be signs of success for those desiring to become master preceptors.

In summary, developing a pharmacy practice rotation requires significant preparation and planning. To be successful, you should design an appropriate curriculum, conduct an effective orientation, assign the student to interesting and relevant responsibilities, and continually evaluate and seek to improve the rotation. While developing, delivering, maintaining, and improving a practice site requires serious preceptor effort, the sacrifice is well worth the satisfaction you receive when your pharmacy intern finishes the rotation inspired to positively impact the profession of pharmacy.

Essential Components of a Continuous Quality Improvement Process for Your Experiential Training Program

There are many definitions of continuous quality improvement (CQI). Here are three definitions from the American Society for Quality, The Delaware Healthcare Association, and the Mental Health Association of Ohio. One of them should apply to almost any education program.

1. "Philosophy and attitude for analyzing capabilities and processes and improving them repeatedly to achieve the objective of customer satisfaction."[12]

2. "Process to continuously make everything better each day. The initiative is customer focused and requires that processes be analyzed, measured, improved and evaluated on an ongoing basis."[13]

3. "An approach to the continuous study and improvement of the processes of providing healthcare services to meet the needs of individuals and others. Synonyms include continuous quality improvement, continuous improvement, organization-wide performance improvement, and total quality management."[14]

The key point that every definition contains is that the process is continuous in developing ways to improve a program. New standards from the Accreditation Council for Pharmacy Education (ACPE) require a continuous quality program for experiential education.

ACPE Guideline 14.6 states,

A quality assurance procedure for all pharmacy practice experiences should be established and implemented to facilitate achievement of stated competencies, provide for feedback, and support standardization, consistency, and inter-rater reliability in assessment of student performance. All practice sites and preceptors should be selected in accordance with quality criteria established and reviewed periodically for quality improvement. The assessment process should incorporate the perspectives of key constituents, such as students, practitioners, prospective employers, and board of pharmacy members.[15]

The ACPE Board of Directors and staff act as judges of the quality of a pharmacy school curriculum. They also expect that each school will have its own standards and ways of assessing curricula and faculty to ensure that minimum educational and program standards are met, such as those described in Guideline 14.6.

• Preceptor Pearls •

The American Society for Quality (www.asq.org) provides resources for continuous improvement strategies.

To meet this guideline, pharmacy school experiential education faculty will approach preceptors and pharmacy or institution leadership to develop and implement educational programs that provide opportunities for students to learn and practice the profession. The expectation will be, in addition to the school requirements for the course, that there will be requirements of the program at the site. The following discussion is meant to spur ideas for development of continuous quality indicators and staff involvement that can increase opportunities for improving quality.

Many colleges of pharmacy have one or more committees to evaluate and assess the curricula and the programs offered. The committee or task force that most likely will affect preceptors is one that functions in the Department of Pharmacy Practice or the Office of Experiential Education. The administration and faculty in the practice department are most concerned with student education at the practice sites and availability of opportunities for students to apply their knowledge. The committee may be called the Continuous Quality Improvement (CQI) committee, or the Experiential Education Programs Assessment (EPAC) committee, or a variety of other names. The responsibilities of this committee are to evaluate and assess practice sites, preceptors, and the program at a site. Members will be looking at technology, the number of people involved in the program, the education of the individuals involved in the program, and opportunities available for student education (Box 6.10).

Box 6.10 • Continuous Quality Improvement—What a School Requires

Site

- Meets accrediting body standards
- Is accessible to students and faculty
- Maintains and advances technology in pharmacy practice
- Maintains and provides technology to students in order to meet the demands of the course (computer, etc.)
- Provides administrative support for student training programs

Preceptor

- Is licensed and meets appropriate State Board standards for providing education to students
- Has a plan for education program to meet needs of students and school
- Has technology available to meet the needs of the college or school of pharmacy
- Has appropriate education and/or experience to provide the opportunities to meet goals and objectives of course maintained by college or school
- Has a contingency plan in place to cover primary preceptor absences
- Is internally motivated to provide educational opportunities
- Is responsive to representative from college or school
- Is involved in professional organizations, community, and/or public health activities, advancing the pharmacy profession

Box 6.10 • Continuous Quality Improvement—What a School Requires (cont'd)

Site Program

- Provides students with multiple opportunities to meet course goals and objectives
- Involves multiple disciplines and/or the community in educational program
- Promotes and incorporates the use of technology for student learning
- Encourages group discussions and peer interaction, which are common among all students
- Provides reflection opportunities for students and preceptors
- Provides access to institution amenities as applicable

These committees take into account assessments from students, assessments from peers, personal interactions with the preceptors at the site, and involvement of preceptors in college or school educational programs. Most schools and colleges have students complete an evaluation form that includes information about the site, and/or the preceptor, and/or the program. The schools then share the information contained in these forms directly with preceptors in a way that provides anonymous feedback. One way a school or faculty member may evaluate the quality of a site is by the interaction of the preceptors with the school as this may be a reflection of how the preceptor also treat the students. Schools do not perceive as quality sites for placement those sites and preceptors who continuously back out of commitments to students. Consider all of the criteria listed in Box 6.10 when developing your educational program for students.

The organization involved in educating students may already have a continuous quality improvement definition in place, which is appropriate to use. If there is not one in place there are several tools from the American Society of Quality that can be used to develop a quality improvement plan. These include the Plan-Do-Check-Act (PDCA), the Six Sigma, and Total Quality Management.

The PDCA model, also called the Deming Cycle, is a workable model for pharmacy education.[16] Implementing the PDCA method of quality assurance is one way to create ongoing quality assessment. The PDCA model can be used at the start of a project or when redefining projects such as educational programs. If your institution has a long standing educational program in place, initiating the PDCA method could provide important information about the program. This model fits well when PLANning for change. The DO component of this tool is to run a test of the change model, or a pilot study. Then CHECK the results of the piloted change. Finally, ACT on the information that has been collected to PLAN the implementation. This cycle will become your ongoing quality improvement model.

Whether you as a preceptor or a team from the pharmacy department decide to develop a quality assurance or continuous improvement program, you should include four elements: peers, students, other healthcare professionals, and the pharmacy school (Box 6.11). Peer assessment comes in the form of those around you who may also work with students or who view your interactions with students. Developing a form similar to one used by human resources departments may provide an indication to you of how others view your performance with students. You should also complete a preceptor self-evaluation each year to see how you think you are doing. Other healthcare providers will be able to provide feedback to you because they have had interactions with students and may have watched your interactions. The feedback they provide may help improve the program logistically or programmatically. Getting feedback from other health professionals may help to draw them into the program either as a preceptor or as an individual who helps you educate the students. Feedback from the college about the educational program is central, but may be provided in various ways.

Box 6.11 • Sources of Assessment and Evaluations of the Site, Preceptor, and Program

- Peer assessment: Provides you with information that you cannot see yourself about the training program and about your actions. Develop an evaluation form such as those used for performance evaluation.

- Student feedback: May provide you with both constructive feedback and comments that may cause you to think twice about taking students, but in the end may help improve the performance of the site and those interacting with students.

- School feedback: May come from student evaluations or from interactions with the school. The feedback may be valuable in helping change the logistics of the rotation at the site, or in changing students' perception of the rotation and the site.

- Feedback from other health professionals: Can provide feedback about student performance as well as logistical assessment of the program provided by your site.

- Patients (if applicable): May discuss a student's performance or how a student was introduced to them. Gather patient evaluations of students, logistics, and what a patient would like to see in a program, whenever possible.

• Preceptor Pearls •

Developing an ongoing quality program for your practice improves outcomes for patients, for students, and for the institution.

Pharmacy school assessment is not always limited to—but may only be provided in—the form of student evaluations. School assessment committees may also provide an annual or periodic review by sending a faculty member to the site to look around and inquire about the program. This assessment by the college or school may just be a phone call to get your input. There are over 100 colleges and schools of pharmacy in the United States and each will operate differently. When seeking to participate with the college program, ask how the school will evaluate you and what quality assurance measures the college has set forth.

Finally, while not all rotations involve direct patient care, those that do could include patients in their quality assurance or improvement measures. Patients can provide a lot of helpful feedback regarding student performance, including how they, as a patient, were treated. Many patients are eager to participate in a program, especially an educational program, in which they feel they are getting one-on-one attention. Some patients may be hesitant to participate, but even those who are not interested can provide feedback on why they do not wish to participate. Consider developing a continuous, quality improvement program as an extension of your practice.

Involving All Pharmacy Staff Members, Other Healthcare Professionals, and Patients

It is important to involve all members of the pharmacy department, not just one individual pharmacist, in student education. Familiarize staff members with students' goals and objectives as well as the roles that everyone will play. Staff involvement can help reduce the workload and stress that often result from the introduction of students into a pharmacy. This is one of the most important aspects in starting or continuing an experiential training program.

• Preceptor Pearls •

Remember that, not only are all members of the pharmacy department involved in student education, you can spread out the workload and lower your stress level by involving other staff.

Anyone who is going to be involved in student education (Table 6.3) is a preceptor in some capacity, and everyone should recognize this fact. It may come in the form of recognition from the college, or the pharmacy, or larger institution. It increases the commitment to the program, and students become more accepting when that recognition exists. Who can be a preceptor is an age-old question, and is defined by the ACPE and many State Boards of Pharmacy. In most instances, a pharmacist should be considered the preceptor of record. However, many other licensed health professionals are considered the preceptor for various types of experiences where pharmacists are not involved full time. Students are going to be in contact with many people who will provide them with various amounts of knowledge, practice of skills, and opportunities for learning. At the very least, the school should recognize pharmacists and technicians in the pharmacy as participating in the program.

• Preceptor Pearls •

Involving other pharmacy staff and other healthcare professionals in the educational programs improves the quality.

Pharmacy technicians often spend a lot of time with students teaching them the technical skills they need to be pharmacists. This is especially true of the IPPEs. Often, students do not view the technician's role as valuable to them; in this case, the primary preceptor should point out the

Table 6.3 • *Responsibilities of Those Involved in Student Education*	
Role	Topics to Teach
Preceptor	• *Logistics of course* • *Rounding* • *Journal clubs* • *Projects* • *Feedback and assessment* • *General practice skills: patient-care or nondirect patient-care oriented* • *Presentations* • *Acclimation to the profession, site, and other healthcare professionals* • *Integration of knowledge and skills in practice*
Other pharmacists	• *General practice skills: patient-care or nondirect patient-care oriented* • *Journal clubs* • *Presentations* • *Acclimation to the profession, site, and other healthcare professionals* • *Integration of knowledge and skills in practice*
Technicians	• *General practice techniques and skills* • *Acclimation to the site* • *Introductions* • *Rules and regulations*
Management/ administrative staff	• *General business and operational/management skills* • *Business rules and regulations* • *Acclimation to the site*
Physicians	• *Precepting* • *Diagnosis of disease* • *Procedures* • *Physical assessment* • *Communication and professional interaction* • *Integration of knowledge and skills in practice* • *Collaboration*
Nursing	• *Logistics* • *Orienting to contents and location of charts* • *Specific patient care* • *Physical assessment, medication administration, and management logistics* • *Collaboration*
Laboratory staff	• *Exposure to the laboratory procedures* • *Lab panels at the site* • *Normal and abnormal results* • *Drugs that interfere with testing*
Patients	• *Development and improvement of communication skills* • *Understanding of disease state outcomes* • *Medications* • *Drug interactions* • *Adherence*

important role the pharmacy technician plays in his or her education. Technicians need to know what their own roles and duties are in student education. The technical staff can educate students in the day-to-day operational skills required in the pharmacy—including filling carts, delivering medications, the IV room function, and the daily ordering processes. For students who have never been in a pharmacy before, assigning them duties with the head technician for a period of time is not unreasonable. Once students have been exposed to the technical duties required, they can move on to the duties of a pharmacist.

All pharmacists and other staff who are going to be involved with students need to understand their own roles in the training as well as the goals and objectives of the students (Box 6.12). It is a good idea to set up an organizational meeting and an annual meeting for those taking responsibility for students. Announce which schools will be sending students. This meeting should address the kind of students who will be assigned to the site. All schools of pharmacy have implemented introductory practice experience courses; consequently, not all students who attend a site for practice skills are in their last year.

Box 6.12 • Guidelines for Involving Others in the Experiential Education Program for Pharmacy Interns

Do

- Involve as many people as possible in the program
- Explain roles and authority to the person you are enlisting to help
- Explain that the students are taking a course
- Discuss the goals and objectives of the course
- Explain the student responsibilities to the site
- Include involved individuals in the orientation program for students
- Schedule their time with students
- Provide a copy of the manual and evaluation tool used by the college
- Get feedback from involved individuals on student performance
- Provide those involved with feedback from students about their performance

Do NOT

- Leave students in the office or work area of anyone who is not involved
- Ask someone to help without providing the list of dos

Plan a course with the pharmacists, technicians, and any other healthcare providers who will be involved in the educational program; involve the college of pharmacy experiential education leadership if necessary. In the end, you should develop a schedule that includes the days and activities as well as who will be providing or overseeing those activities.

In a community setting, it is mostly the pharmacists and technicians involved in the educational programs, but they do not have to be the only contacts for students. Ask physicians who work closely with the pharmacy if students can spend some time in their offices. If the community setting is a chain store, include the district manager in the educational functions. Many of the district managers already precept student rotations, and they enjoy the opportunity to mentor students.

There are many other settings where students are educated as well: the pharmaceutical industry mail order companies, veterinary practice settings, home infusion services, and nursing homes. Various professionals and technical staff at each of these sites can become involved with student education.

Involving many people in student programs (especially people who often come into contact with students) is good practice, even if for logistical purposes only. The more that people know about pharmacy education, the better they will accept the students, and the greater the likelihood is of having a quality educational program that will enable student success.

• Preceptor Pearls •

Experiential education is not just an opportunity for preceptors, but for an entire pharmacy staff, to improve practice and advance the profession.

Continuous quality improvement should not be a scary process. It is a process that requires planning, integration of assessment, and a team effort. When putting together an experiential education program, ask peers, staff, and other health professionals to become involved. Discern how they would like be involved before you start planning and integrate them into the plan. Have a plan in place for educational opportunities and continuous improvement weeks before students arrive. Make sure that information on the program is both outgoing and incoming. Gather assessment often and from multiple sources. Learn from the information gathered and improve and build your program with each student you precept.

References

1. Accreditation Council for Pharmacy Education. Accreditation standards and guidelines for the professional program in pharmacy leading to the doctor of pharmacy degree. Available at: http://www.acpe-accredit.org/pdf/ACPE_Revised_PharmD_Standards_Adopted_Jan152006.pdf. Accessed April 1, 2008.

2. Chisholm MA, DiPiro JT, Fagan SC. An innovative introductory pharmacy practice experience model. *Am J Pharm Educ.* 2003;67:171–8.

3. Turner CJ, Altiere R, Clark L, et al. An interdisciplinary introductory pharmacy practice experience course. *Am J Pharm Educ.* 2004;68:10.

4. Turner CJ, Ellis S, Giles J, et al. An introductory pharmacy practice experience emphasizing student-administered vaccinations. *Am J Pharm Educ.* 2007;71:3.

5. Irby DM, Wilkerson L. *Teaching rounds:* Teaching when time is limited. *Br Med J.* 2008;336:384–7.

6. Kaufman DM. ABC of learning and teaching in medicine: applying educational theory in practice. *Br Med J.* 2003;326:213–6.

7. Papadakis MA, Teherani A, Banach MA, et al. Disciplinary action by medical boards and prior behavior in medical school. *N Engl J Med.* 2005;353:2673–82.

8. Hamilton KE. Presenting to different types of learners. Available at: http://webhome.idirect.com/~kehamilt/spklearn. Accessed April 2008.

9. Blanchard K, Johnson S. *The One Minute Manager.* New York, NY: HarperCollins Publishers; 1982.

10. Beck DE, O'Sullivan PS, Boh LE. Increasing the accuracy of observer ratings by enhancing cognitive processing skills. *Am J Pharm Educ.* 1995;59:228–35.

11. University of Texas at Austin College of Pharmacy. Course syllabus for Advanced Pharmacy Practice Rotations. May 2008.

12. American Society for Quality. American Society for Quality glossary. Available at: http://www.asq.org/glossary/c.html. Accessed May 2008.

13. Delaware Healthcare Association. Delaware Healthcare Association glossary of healthcare terms and acronyms. Available at: http://www.deha.org/Glossary/GlossaryC.htm. Accessed May 2008.

14. Mental Health Association. Available at: http://www.mh.state.oh.us/. Accessed May 2008.

15. Accreditation Council for Pharmacy Education. Introduction to the professional degree program accreditation process. Available at: http://www.acpe-accredit.org/deans/accreditation.asp. Accessed May 2008.

16. American Society for Quality. Plan-Do-Check-Act Cycle. Available at: http://www.asq.org/learn-about-quality/project-planning-tools/overview/pdca-cycle.html. Accessed May 2008.

In civilized life, law floats in a sea of ethics.
Earl Warren

Chapter 7

Law and Ethics in Experiential Training

Vikki Jill Polk, Diane B. Ginsburg

Chapter Outline

Learning Objectives

- Describe each of the six common requirements for pharmacists to become preceptors within their respective states.
- Discuss liability issues for preceptors.
- Understand the Code of Ethics for pharmacists and explain how it applies to experiential training.
- Define the Health Insurance Portability and Accountability Act (HIPAA) and describe how it applies to experiential training programs.

The curriculum in pharmacy education today is divided almost evenly between didactic and experiential learning. Students must devote many hours toward hands-on learning in order to achieve their pharmacy degree. Pharmacy preceptors willing to train and teach students must adhere to specific guidelines in order to supervise pharmacist interns. In addition, preceptors must also follow ethical and HIPAA guidelines when directing interns. This chapter will review requirements for preceptors.

Pharmacy Rules and Regulations: State Board of Pharmacy Requirements for Preceptors

A preceptor plays a significant role in the training and development of future pharmacist practitioners. Most states mandate that hours worked in a pharmacy must be under the direct supervision of a pharmacist who is certified as a preceptor, if those hours are to be counted towards graduating from a school of pharmacy. This requirement does not necessarily apply to hours that students must complete to satisfy degree requirements of their respective academic program. It is not uncommon for pharmacist interns to complete a rotation during their experiential program and be supervised by a physician or other healthcare provider.

• Preceptor Pearls •

States vary widely in their requirements for preceptors, but they usually include some combination of the following: predetermined length of practice, application, approval and/or certification, a training seminar, and good legal standing.

For certification as a preceptor, most states require that a pharmacist be licensed and have at least one year of experience in his or her respective practice setting. Some states recognize pharmacy residency program training and allow pharmacy residents to apply for preceptor certification during their residency (e.g., Texas will allow a pharmacist who has been in an American Society of Health-System Pharmacists (ASHP) accredited residency for at least six months to serve as a preceptor if all other requirements are met).

Only a few states require some form of preceptor education as part of the initial certification process. To maintain preceptor status, preceptors are required to complete additional hours of preceptor-specific education to maintain their certification. In some states, this continuing education is tied to the licensure renewal cycle. Some colleges require that preceptors complete continuing education specific to their program prior to their certification as preceptors. Many colleges and schools offer annual preceptor education conferences as well as partnering with state professional associations to provide preceptor training.

Each state has its own requirements regarding the ratio of preceptors to interns. Most states limit this ratio to one-to-one when providing direct patient care activities. In some states, colleges of pharmacy may apply for an exemption to this rule to allow for an expansion of the ratio. They might need exemption in nontraditional practice settings or in situations where the hours completed by an intern are for satisfying degree requirements rather than for licensure.

The supervision and teaching of future practitioners is a large responsibility for preceptors. The purpose of the internship program is for students to learn the proper way to practice pharmacy while abiding by all laws and rules that govern pharmacy practice. Licenses must be in good standing in order for pharmacists to supervise pharmacy students. Unfortunately, things can happen in a pharmacy that can result in disciplinary action against the pharmacy and/or pharmacist's license even if he or she were not directly responsible. Even though there may not have been any malicious intent on the part of the pharmacist preceptor, a pharmacy and pharmacist who are the subjects of a board-imposed penalty should not precept students until the disciplinary action has been resolved and the licenses have been returned to good standing. Some states do allow pharmacists to petition the board to have their preceptor certification reinstated at an earlier time. In this case, it is up to the individual board of pharmacy to render this decision. Pharmacy board requirements for preceptors by state are listed in Table 7.1.

Licensure

Licensure is not a section in Table 7.1 since pharmacists are already required to be licensed by the board or regulatory agent of the particular state in which they will be serving as preceptors. Every state has deemed pharmacists to be preceptors because they are licensed pharmacists and have met the other requirements. Most often it is noted that the pharmacist must be in good standing. Some states do not require preceptors in the areas of drug research within a pharmacy school or industry to be licensed pharmacists. An exception to this would be pharmacists practicing in federal facilities who are only required to have a current license in at least one state. Pharmacists practicing in any of the military branches, the Veteran's Administration, or the Bureau of Prisons are only required to be licensed in one state and may practice pharmacy in any facility regardless of location. Federal laws, not individual state laws, have jurisdiction in these facilities.

Table 7.1 • *Board of Pharmacy Requirements for Preceptors*

State	Length of Practice	Complete Application	Approval/ Certification	Training Seminar	Legal Standing
Alabama-[1]	2 y-	Yes-	Approval	Yes-	No
Alaska[2]	n/a	No	n/a	No	No
Arizona[a,3]	1 y	Yes	Approval	No	Yes-
Arkansas[a,4]	1 y	Yes	Certification	No	Yes-
California[5]	n/a	No	n/a	No	Yes-
Colorado[a,6]	2 y	Yes-	Both-	No	5 y
Connecticut[7]	n/a	No	n/a	No	No
Delaware[8]	2 y-	No	n/a	No	No
D.C.[a,9]	n/a	No	Approval	No	Yes
Florida[10]	n/a	No	n/a	No	Yes-
Georgia[11]	n/a	No	n/a	No	No
Hawaii[12]	n/a	No	n/a	No	No
Idaho[13]	n/a	No	n/a	No	No
Illinois[14]	n/a	No	n/a	No	No
Indiana[a,15]	n/a	No	n/a	No	No
Iowa[16]	n/a	No	n/a	No	Yes
Kansas[17]	2 y	No	Approval	No	No
Kentucky[a,18]	1 y-	No	Certification	No	No
Louisiana[19]	n/a	No	Certification	No	No
Maine[20]	2 y	No	n/a	No	No
Maryland[a,21]	n/a	No	n/a	No	Yes-
Massachusetts[22]	1 y-	No	Approval	No	No
Michigan[23]	1 y	Yes-	Approval	No	5 y
Minnesota[24]	4,000 h	Yes-	Approval	Yes	Yes
Mississippi[25]	n/a	No	n/a	No	Yes
Missouri[26]	n/a	No	Approval	No	Yes
Montana[27]	2 y	Yes-	Approval	No	3 y
Nebraska[28]	n/a	No	n/a	No	No
Nevada[29]	n/a	No	n/a	No	No
New Hampshire[30]	n/a	No	n/a	No	No
New Jersey[31]	2 y	Yes-	Certification	No	Yes-
New Mexico[32]	1 y	Yes	Certification	No	3 y
New York[33]	1 y	No	n/a	No	No
North Carolina[a,34]	n/a	No	n/a	No	Yes-
North Dakota[35]	n/a	No	n/a	No	Yes
Ohio[36]	n/a	No	n/a	No	Yes
Oklahoma[a,37]	1 y	Yes-	Certification	No	Yes
Oregon[38]	1 y	Yes	Approval	No	No
Pennsylvania[3,9]	n/a	Yes	n/a	No	Yes
Rhode Island[40]	n/a	No	n/a	No	No
South Carolina[41]	n/a	No	n/a	No	No
South Dakota[42]	n/a	Yes	n/a	No	No
Tennessee[43]	n/a	No	n/a	No	No
Texas[44]	1 y-	Yes	Both	Yes-	Yes

Table 7.1 • *Board of Pharmacy Requirements for Preceptors (cont'd)*

State	Length of Practice	Complete Application	Approval/ Certification	Training Seminar	Legal Standing
Utah[a,45]	*2 y-*	*No*	*n/a*	*No*	*Yes*
Vermont[46]	*1 y*	*No*	*Approval*	*No*	*Yes*
Virginia[47]	*n/a*	*No*	*n/a*	*No*	*No*
Washington[48]	*1 y-*	*No*	*Certification*	*Yes-*	*Yes-*
West Virginia[49]	*n/a*	*No*	*n/a*	*No*	*No*
Wisconsin[50]	*n/a*	*No*	*n/a*	*No*	*No*
Wyoming[51]	*2 y-*	*Yes-*	*Both*	*No*	*No*

[1] Alabama: http://www.albop.com/.

[2] Alaska: http://www.dced.state.ak.us/occ/ppha.htm.

[3] Arizona: http://www.pharmacy.state.az.us/pdfs/PRECEPTOR.pdf.

[4] Arkansas: http://www.arkansas.gov/asbp/pdf/preceptor_application.pdf.

[5] California: http://www.pharmacy.ca.gov/intern_preceptor_manual.htm#appendix_c; California Code of Regulations, Chapter 17, Title 16, Section 1726: http://www.pharmacy.ca.gov/rph_licensee.htm#preceptor.

[6] Colorado: http://www.dora.state.co.us/pharmacy/int/INTmanual.pdf and http://www.dora.state.co.us/Pharmacy/int/PHApreceptor.pdf .

[7] Connecticut: No information available for this state.

[8] Delaware: http://www.dpr.delaware.gov/boards/pharmacy/documents/PRACTICAL_EXPERIENCE_PROGRAM_FOR_PHARMACY_PRECEPTORS_AND_INTERNS.doc.

[9] District of Columbia: http://dchealth.dc.gov/doh/frames.asp?doc=/doh/lib/doh/prof_license/services/pdffile/pharmacy/MunicipalPharmacistsRegulations.pdf&dohNav=|34535|.

[10] Florida: https://www.flrules.org/gateway/RuleNo.asp?ID=64B16-26.400.

[11] Georgia: http://www.sos.state.ga.us/acrobat/examboards/pharmacy/intern_2002.pdf.

[12] Hawaii: http://hawaii.gov/dcca/areas/pvl/boards/pharmacy/application_publications/.

[13] Idaho: http://www3.idaho.gov/oasis/H0390.html.

[14] Illinois: http://www.ilga.gov/commission/jcar/admincode/068/068013300000200R.html.

[15] Indiana: http://www.in.gov/pla/4418.htm.

[16] Iowa: http://www.state.ia.us/ibpe/pharmacists/preceptor.html.

[17] Kansas: http://www.accesskansas.org/pharmacy/leg.html.

[18] Kentucky: http://pharmacy.ky.gov/professional/interninfo.htm.

[19] Louisiana: http://www.labp.com.

[20] Maine: http://www.maine.gov/sos/cec/rules/02/392/392.doc.

[21] Maryland: http://www.dhmh.state.md.us/pharmacyboard/faq/index.htm.

[22] Massachusetts: http://www.mass.gov/Eeohhs2/docs/dph/regs/247cmr002.pdf.

[23] Michigan: http://www.michigan.gov/documents/mdch_pharm_preceptor_app_123564_7.pdf.

[24] Minnesota: http://www.phcybrd.state.mn.us/forms/preceptorapp.pdf.

[25] Mississippi: http://www.mbp.state.ms.us/mbop/Pharmacy.nsf/webpageedit/RegulationsLN_regdb_Requirement/$FILE/Requirement.pdf?OpenElement.

[26] Missouri: http://www.sos.mo.gov/adrules/csr/current/20csr/20c2220-2.pdf.

[27] Montana: http://www.discoveringmontana.com/dli/bsd/license/bsd_boards/pha_board/rules.asp#6.

[28] Nebraska: http://www.sos.state.ne.us/rules-and-regs/regsearch/Rules/Health_and_Human_Services_System/Title-175/Chapter-8.pdf.

[29] Nevada: http://www.leg.state.nv.us/Register/2003Register/R019-03P.pdf.

[30] New Hampshire: http://www.gencourt.state.nh.us/rsa/html/XXX/318/318-18.htm.

[31] New Jersey: http://www.state.nj.us/oag/ca/laws/pharmregs.pdf.

[32] New Mexico: http://www.rld.state.nm.us/Pharmacy/PDFs/PRECEPTOR%20APPLICATION.pdf.

[33] New York: http://www.op.nysed.gov/pharm4.pdf.

[34] North Carolina: http://www.ncbop.org/Forms%20and%20Applications%20-%20Pharmacists/Internship Registration.pdf.

[35] North Dakota: http://www.nodakpharmacy.com/NDBP/law/2008LegislativeChanges.pdf.

[36] Ohio: http://pharmacy.ohio.gov/intrnshp-030201.htm.

[37] Oklahoma: http://www.ok.gov/OSBP/documents/law05.pdf.

[38] Oregon: http://arcweb.sos.state.or.us/rules/OARS_800/OAR_855/855_031.html.

[39] Pennsylvania: http://www.pacode.com/secure/data/049/chapter27/s27.26.html and http://www.dos.state.pa.us/bpoa/lib/bpoa/20/phabd/preceptor0703.pdf.

[40] Rhode Island: http://www2.sec.state.ri.us/dar/regdocs/released/pdf/DOH/5042.pdf.

[41] South Carolina: http://www.scstatehouse.net/code/t40c043.htm.

[42] South Dakota: http://legis.state.sd.us/statutes/DisplayStatute.aspx?Type=Statute&Statute=36-11-25.

[43] Tennessee: http://www.state.tn.us/sos/rules/1140/1140-02.pdf.

[44] Texas: http://www.tsbp.state.tx.us/files_Word/CERT-PRECEPTOR.doc.

Table 7.1 • *Board of Pharmacy Requirements for Preceptors (cont'd)*

[45]Utah: http://www.dopl.utah.gov/laws/58-17b.pdf.
[46]Vermont: http://vtprofessionals.org/opr1/pharmacists/forms/rxrules.pdf.
[47]Virginia: http://www.dhp.state.va.us/pharmacy/leg/Pharmacy%20Law%202007-8-23-07.doc.
[48]Washington State: http://apps.leg.wa.gov/WAC/default.aspx?cite=246-858-070, http://apps.leg.wa.gov/WAC/default.aspx?cite=246-858-060.
[49]West Virginia: http://www.wvbop.com.
[50]Wisconsin: http://drl.wi.gov/dept/forms/fm2539.pdf.
[51]Wyoming: http://pharmacyboard.state.wy.us/laws/Pharmacy_Act.pdf.

Length of Practice

Only 21 states require that a pharmacist have practiced for a specific length of time before they can precept students, and the length of practice is typically the 1–2 years immediately before becoming a preceptor. Some states specify a number of years (e.g., in Arkansas, 2 years), but others require a certain number of hours practicing (e.g., in Minnesota, 4,000 hours with 2,000 of the 4,000 hours within the state).

Complete Application

Fourteen states require pharmacists to complete an application before they can be considered preceptors. These forms are typically located on the website of the board or regulatory agent. This application usually registers pharmacists as preceptors for the particular state in which they are applying.

Approval and Certification

The board of pharmacy or regulatory agent of a state will grant preceptor approval to pharmacists who meet the requirements needed to precept students. Twenty-one states require certification to become preceptors, and some states require pharmacists to be both approved and certified. It is common for a preceptor to be certified for a specified number of years, after which they must apply for recertification, which sometimes involves an exam and fees. Many of the states that require certification also require that the certificate be displayed in a conspicuous location.

Training Seminar

Very few states (i.e., Alabama, Minnesota, Texas, and Washington) have a required board-approved preceptor-training seminar for applicants. These seminars are required for initial approval and then as often as the state deems it necessary to meet requirements, ranging from 2–5 years. Attendance of this training program must be completed again when pharmacists' current licenses are to be renewed.

Legal Standing

Most state boards of pharmacy and regulatory agents do not cite good legal standing as a requirement for preceptor applicants. This means that they must be in compliance with the law and must not have violated any laws or statutes related to the practice of pharmacy. Only 23 states document observation of law observance in their requirements. Most states list "good standing with the Board" after licensure requirements, and this can often be interpreted as good legal compliance with the rules and regulations of the state's pharmacy laws. However, it is best to give an exact legal compliance time frame, so that expectations are clearly projected. Legal standing refers to either the specific time period of law observance or if law observance was noted for a particular state. States might require that a pharmacist have an unrestricted pharmacist's license or apply for and receive special permission to become a preceptor if they are involved in any legal issues.

The requirements for pharmacists to become preceptors vary widely from state to state, with some states having unique requirements (Box 7.1). Being a licensed pharmacist is the only criterion that all states have in common. Table 7.1 makes it apparent that some states have highly structured procedures that are expected of pharmacists wanting to become preceptors. It is important to fully research the requirements of your state to ensure you follow all necessary procedures.

Box 7.1 • Examples of Unique State Requirements

- The Arizona State Board of Pharmacy requires that a pharmacist either be approved by the board or hold a faculty position that is part of the experiential training program of an approved college or school of pharmacy. A pharmacist must "be a full-time pharmacist in a pharmacy which currently holds a Class A rating indicated by the 'Inspection Sheet' for pharmacists outlined by the State Board of Pharmacy." The applicant must also complete a preceptor requirements and responsibilities test that was developed and administered by the board or board representatives. It is required that one preceptor from an intern site be a member of an "appropriate" national pharmaceutical organization.

- In Arkansas, each individual preceptor is required to be a member of a professional state organization and attend one professional meeting during the previous calendar year. Regulation 01-00-0007 specifies fees that are required during the renewal process that takes place every 2 years and requires a new application.

- In the District of Columbia, pharmacists wanting to be preceptors must take the "Oath of Preceptor," which is as follows: "I submit that I shall answer all questions concerning the training of a pharmacy intern under my supervision truthfully to the best of my knowledge and belief and that the training I provide will be predominately related to the practice of pharmacy as required by law."

- Pharmacists wanting to be board-approved preceptors in Indiana must include "a detailed description of the proposed practical experience program with respect to time, place, duties, responsibilities, and supervision; and the name of the person responsible for supervising the experience."

- To be preceptors in Kentucky, pharmacists must submit a written request.

- In Maine, preceptors are assigned by the pharmacist-in-charge at a site for interns.

- In North Carolina, if preceptors supervise at least 400 hours of intern experience, the board will grant them 5 hours of continuing education credits.

- In Ohio, a preceptor can be a pharmacist or a "person who is of good moral character and is qualified to direct the approved experience in the area approved by the director of internship pursuant to paragraph (D) of rule 4729 3 05 of the Administrative Code."

Box 7.1 • Examples of Unique State Requirements (cont'd)

- Oklahoma requires pharmacists to take a preceptor exam that is prepared by the board and pay a fee. Verbal examination is also part of the application process.

- Utah applicants must provide proof of meeting the requirements for continuing education for the 2 years prior to license renewal. "Applicants must also subscribe to and abide by the Code of Ethics of the American Pharmacists' Association."

- In Oregon, nonpharmacists preceptors can be designated to supervise interns with the Board's approval.

- In Wisconsin, preceptors can contact the pharmacy school directly instead of registering through the Wisconsin State Board of Pharmacy.

• Preceptor Pearls •

Use Table 7.1 or do an online search to find out all of the requirements for your state.

Liability Issues for Preceptors

The training of future pharmacists is a rewarding experience for most preceptors. Students are eager after many years of training to function as licensed practitioners and provide direct patient care. Many students, when they enter the final year of their program, are very mature and appear ready to undertake the responsibilities of licensed pharmacists. The important thing to remember is that, although they may seem ready to function as licensed practitioners, they are not licensed. The responsibility of all student actions rests with the preceptor's license.

• Preceptor Pearls •

Remind students that you, as their preceptor, are *ultimately responsible* for everything they do and that your license could be disciplined for failure to be in compliance with appropriate laws and rules.

Most colleges of pharmacy understand the huge responsibility that preceptors have when they are supervising students. Preceptors not only have to worry about their actions (and in some cases, the actions of their staff if they are the pharmacist-in-charge or in another supervisory role), but they also have to worry about the actions of their students. Most students do not intentionally try to make an error; however, the nature of their learning process lends itself to the fact that students are going to make mistakes. Preceptors are ultimately responsible for any errors made by students. This reinforces the importance of checking all work completed by students.

Most programs require that students purchase liability insurance prior to starting their rotations.

These policies, which range between $10.00 and $20.00, only cover activities that the students perform. These policies are not the same as the malpractice insurance that most licensed pharmacists carry.

Ethical Aspects of Precepting Students

The practice of pharmacy is governed by a strict Code of Ethics (Box 7.2). This code has been endorsed by virtually all facets of pharmacy and reflects the nature of practice today, a cooperative relationship between pharmacists, other healthcare providers, and patients. As pharmacists, we think of ethics and this code as the way pharmacy should be practiced; for most of us, this is the way we practice.

Box 7.2 • Code of Ethics for Pharmacists[a]

Preamble

Pharmacists are health professionals who assist individuals in making the best use of medications. This code, prepared and supported by pharmacists, is intended to state publicly the principles that form the fundamental basis of the roles and responsibilities of pharmacists. These principles, based on moral obligations and virtues, are established to guide pharmacists in relationships with patients, health professionals, and society.

I. A pharmacist respects the covenantal relationship between the patient and pharmacist.

Considering the patient-pharmacist relationship as a covenant means that a pharmacist has moral obligations in response to the gift of trust received from society. In return for this gift, a pharmacist promises to help individuals achieve optimum benefit from their medications, to be committed to their welfare, and to maintain their trust.

II. A pharmacist promotes the good of every patient in a caring, compassionate, and confidential manner.

A pharmacist places concern for the well being of the patient at the center of professional practice. In doing so, a pharmacist considers needs stated by the patient as well as those defined by health science. A pharmacist is dedicated to protecting the dignity of the patient. With a caring attitude and a compassionate spirit, a pharmacist focuses on serving the patient in a private and confidential manner.

III. A pharmacist respects the autonomy and dignity of each patient.

A pharmacist promotes the right of self-determination and recognizes individual self-worth by encouraging patients to participate in decisions about their health. A pharmacist communicates with patients in terms that are understandable. In all cases, a pharmacist respects personal and cultural differences among patients.

IV. A pharmacist acts with honesty and integrity in professional relationships.

A pharmacist has a duty to tell the truth and to act with conviction of conscience. A pharmacist avoids discriminatory practices, behavior or work conditions that impair professional judgment, and actions that compromise dedication to the best interests of patients.

Box 7.2 • Code of Ethics for Pharmacists[a] (cont'd)

V. A pharmacist maintains professional competence.

A pharmacist has a duty to maintain knowledge and abilities as new medications, devices, and technologies become available and as health information advances.

VI. A pharmacist respects the values and abilities of colleagues and other health professionals.

When appropriate, a pharmacist asks for the consultation of colleagues or other health professionals or refers the patient. A pharmacist acknowledges that colleagues and other health professionals may differ in the beliefs and values they apply to the care of the patient.

VII. A pharmacist serves individual, community, and societal needs.

The primary obligation of a pharmacist is to individual patients. However, the obligations of a pharmacist may at times extend beyond the individual to the community and society. In these situations, the pharmacist recognizes the responsibilities that accompany these obligations and acts accordingly.

VIII. A pharmacist seeks justice in the distribution of health resources.

When health resources are allocated, a pharmacist is fair and equitable, balancing the needs of patients and society."

[a]Adopted by the membership of the American Pharmacists Association, October 27, 1994. This applies to the Code of Ethics.

Source: American Pharmacists Association. Code of Ethics for Pharmacists. Washington, DC: American Pharmacists Association; 1997.

The preceptor's role is multifold. Preceptors are teachers, mentors, coaches, references, and role models. The future of the profession, our students, looks up to us for guidance, information, and to mirror our actions. These reasons reinforce the importance of ethical behavior and a review of the code that governs our practice.

• Preceptor Pearls •

Review the Code of Ethics with your students and discuss how it impacts your practice.

Many students remember receiving and/or reciting the Code of Ethics during the white coat ceremony that is usually held during new student orientation. As novices they blindly recite the words, not truly understanding the significance behind them. Many will not think to pull out this document until something happens and they are reminded of this code. As preceptors, it is essential that students see you uphold and abide by this code. Review and discuss with your students what the Code of Ethics means to you as a pharmacist and how you demonstrate this in your practice.

As important as this code is to practice, it is equally important that preceptors and their staff treat students with respect and dignity. Many issues come into play when precepting students: demands of the work place, staff needs, knowledge base of the students, and generational differences. Today's students can use automated databases and computers more comfortably than a print textbook. They have been taught drug information using an integrated approach rather than by discipline (e.g., chemistry, pharmacology, clinical application). For some tenured practitioners, this presents both an opportunity and a challenge. The opportunity is one in which students can teach preceptors and expose them to the benefits of their education. The challenge for some preceptors is resistance to a new model for pharmacy practice and the way students are being taught. Preceptors need to embrace the generational nuances that today's students bring to the practice environment and respect the methods by which students access and retrieve information.

Patient Confidentiality and HIPAA

The issue of patient confidentiality was heightened as a result of privacy laws enacted by the federal government. The Health Insurance Portability and Accountability Act (HIPAA) increased the level of due diligence that healthcare providers must exercise to ensure confidentiality of patient Protected Health Information (PHI). Pharmacies and all healthcare institutions have implemented safeguards and protective measures, including training of staff, to ensure protection of PHI.

Most colleges and schools of pharmacy have incorporated HIPAA information in pharmacy jurisprudence courses as part of their discussion of federal law. In addition, HIPAA and privacy issues are discussed prior to the beginning of experiential training for most programs and included in course syllabi for the internship. This does not preclude the HIPAA training requirements of the individual practice site. Students may be expected to complete HIPAA training for each rotation if they are completed at different institutions. A review of HIPAA and privacy rules should be included as part of the orientation to the practice site and conducted during the beginning of the rotation experience.

Summary

Precepting students can be a very rewarding experience for pharmacists. A good preceptor must balance the needs of their practice and patients while teaching students. Preceptors must follow and adhere to all applicable laws and regulations when precepting students. Not only will this ensure that pharmacy is being practiced in a legal and ethical manner, the preceptor establishes him or herself as an effective role model when practicing in this manner.

There is incredible liberation in realizing you can change the world simply by changing your perception.

Deepak Chopra, MD

Chapter 8

Teaching Students About Cultural, Social, and Economic Issues Affecting Modern Healthcare

Lourdes M. Cuéllar, Nicanora C. Cuéllar, Dehuti A. Pandya, Michael Piñón

Chapter Outline

Learning Objectives

- Define diversity and describe the value of the diversity of our student population.
- Demonstrate understanding and appreciate the value of working in a culturally diverse environment.
- Teach students the importance of integrating values and beliefs into their daily practice.
- Describe how our own biases or stereotypes can impact our ability to be effective preceptors.
- Explain how culture can shape a person's attitude towards health and healing and how this may impact health outcomes.
- Define health disparity and identify factors that contribute to health disparities.
- Identify legislative changes that have augmented or diminished access to healthcare.
- Describe how recent economic trends have limited access to healthcare.
- Recognize that not having healthcare insurance can be financially devastating for individuals of all income levels.
- Recognize recent economic trends that have curtailed access to healthcare.
- Distinguish employer benefit decisions that are escalating consumer healthcare expenses.
- List populations that are more vulnerable to having inadequate access to health services.
- Define health literacy, and describe its impact on a patient's heath status.
- Demonstrate tools that preceptors and students can use to identify patients with low health literacy skills and to address problems.
- Define culture and cultural competency, and explain the importance of providing culturally competent care.

"Culture is a pattern of learned beliefs, values, and behavior that are shared within a group; it includes language, styles of communication, practices, customs, and views on roles and relationships. We all belong to more than one culture, which may, for example, be social, professional, or religious; the concept goes beyond race, ethnic background, and country of origin. Culture shapes the way we approach our world and affects interactions between patients and clinicians."[1]

Preceptors can effectively teach their students, directly and through role modeling, the knowledge and skills needed to be able to provide services that are appropriate for a diverse patient population. Even a seasoned preceptor must continue to learn and maintain cultural competence skills. This chapter will provide some basic information about social and economic issues relating to healthcare, including access to care, health literacy, and cultural competency. This information will help preceptors to enhance the students' understanding, knowledge, and skills relating to the influence of cultural and social factors on healthcare. By becoming aware of causal factors that could be eliminated or modified and application of appropriate knowledge and skills, we can improve the health status of all our patients.

Effectively Precepting a Diverse Student Population

In the book, *Building a House for Diversity*, R. Roosevelt Thomas, Jr. states that although race and ethnicity are the most obvious components of culture, there are many factors that shape a person's values, ideas, attitudes, and experiences.[2] These include age, gender, disability, sexual orientation, level of education, income, preferred language, urban versus rural location, native versus foreign-born status, customs, beliefs, and practices. An appreciation of the diversity of our pharmacy students by healthcare organizations and preceptors is especially important today as health systems and healthcare practitioners must respond to an increasing racially and ethnically diverse patient population.

A quick review of the demographic statistics of today's pharmacy students indicate that the portrait of our future practitioners differs significantly from what it was even 10 years ago. Today, there are far more females among pharmacy students, and many schools are admitting students (in some cases greater than 30%) with prior degrees, including advanced degrees. In addition, many of the current students are older than the average college student. Likewise, the cultural or ethnic diversity of pharmacy students is significant in many areas of the U.S. However, the diversity of our pharmacy graduates does not match the growing diverse demographics of the U.S. population. The chance of the composition of the healthcare workforce in the U.S. reflecting the diversity of our population in the near future is low. The Census Bureau's 2006 American Community Survey, states that African Americans, Hispanics, and Native Americans now comprise 28% of the U.S. population.[3] However, African Americans, Hispanics, and Native Americans make up a significantly smaller percentage of the student body in colleges and schools of pharmacy in contrast to their representation within the general U.S. population. Of the total number of doctor of pharmacy degrees conferred as first professional degrees in 2006, only 7.4% were earned by African Americans, 4.2% by Hispanics, and 0.4% by Native Americans.[4]

Today, organizational focus has turned toward cultural awareness, or valuing differences. The Institute of Medicine's (IOM) report, *In the Nation's Compelling Interest: Ensuring Diversity in the Healthcare Workforce,* states that increasing racial and ethnic diversity among healthcare professionals is a very important aspect of providing healthcare because evidence suggests that diversity is associated with improved access to care for racial and ethnic minorities.[5] In addition, it provides for greater patient choice in providers, improved patient satisfaction, better patient-clinician communication, and better educational experiences for health profession students.

Preceptors should be aware that culture greatly influences how students view their entire world, whether they are at school, at home, or completing an experiential rotation. You may notice differences among students in such areas as the generally accepted roles for women and men, the importance of the individual versus the family or community, the role of religion in everyday life, modesty in dress, body language, personal interactions, and boundaries regarding eye contact and personal space. Culture also affects how students may deal with critically ill patients and issues surrounding death and dying patients. Students may bring with them their own history or beliefs regarding folk wisdom and common sense compared to formal education and scientific knowledge. The preceptor should thoughtfully inquire about student beliefs regarding illness versus wellness and holistic approach to health (mind, body, spirit) versus western medicine. As we move further toward evidence-based medicine, the need for alternative therapies and their benefits will go under even greater scrutiny and potentially could be ignored or dismissed, making an understanding of cultural diversity even more important.

Preceptors should also recognize their own biases or perceived stereotypes. Do you interact with students in ways that manifest double standards? Do you undervalue comments made by students whose English is accented or who appear foreign? It is very important to avoid ethnocentrism, in which we believe our own culture and way of doing things are the best. Preceptors need to acknowledge and accept that cultural differences exist and may impact their interactions with students. It is important to understand that incorporating the strengths of many cultures enhances the capacity of the whole group. Likewise, the preceptor should recognize that diversity within cultures is as important as diversity between cultures, and as preceptors and educators, we need to value diversity.

The most important concept to keep in mind is that teaching for diversity means teaching to each individual student. One of the greatest challenges you face is modifying your teaching or precepting style to meet the different learning styles of each student. By taking an interest in the students' experiences, interests, beliefs, and goals, you take the most important step in making the students feel that they will succeed on your rotation.

• Preceptor Pearls •

- Become acquainted with your students individually; try to understand their interests, beliefs, and values. Do this on day one of the practice experience.

- Learn every student's name and the name by which he/she prefers to be called, and use that name. If you are not sure, ask for the correct pronunciation.

- Try to anticipate and acknowledge issues of sexuality, religion, or other values when you give projects or assignments.

- Introduce controversial topics in impersonal or nonjudgmental ways.

- Balance practical problem-solving techniques with fundamental methods.

- Do not overlook capable but quiet students; give male and female students equal attention when mentoring and when providing feedback.

- Treat students as individuals, not as representatives of their gender or ethnicity.

- Do not assume that there is a collective identity minority students share.

- Do not make assumptions regarding a student's language capabilities based on ethnic background. (e.g., a student with a Hispanic last name may not necessarily read, speak, or understand Spanish).

- Do not assume all students are heterosexual; respond firmly to inappropriate remarks.

- Take advantage of life experiences as well as the different perspectives that older students bring to the experiential rotation.

- Remember that any student may be dealing with children, mortgages, jobs, marriages, or divorces while they study to become a pharmacist.

- Assume that students hold different religious beliefs. Accommodate students' important religious holidays. Allow for them in planning the student schedule.

- If you have a student with a physical disability or challenge, ask the student privately if there is anything you can do to facilitate learning. Adapt to the student's need without lowering your usual course standards.

- Assume that certain topics may affect some students personally, for example, dealing with illness and disease.

- Monitor your own behavior in responding to students.

- Remember, you teach what you are. Your training style reflects your knowledge, interests, and beliefs.

Remember as a preceptor you are a role model to your students. Share with your students your own experiences and process of developing awareness of the role of gender, recognition of sexual orientation, race, and ethnic stereotypes and issues. Help students understand the value of a diverse perspective in their future professional lives. Use examples from your own life and practice.

Healthcare practitioners and students need to learn the value of a culturally diverse environment, experience culture and gender differences, and appreciate the value of diversity in their daily decision-making process. Teach students the importance of integrating values and beliefs into the daily operations of their practice. Preceptors can exemplify this cultural awareness in their daily practice while interacting with their colleagues, other healthcare providers, and patients. This is integral to the cultural proficiency process. Reach out to students who are different in race, culture, or gender. Teach all students how to navigate successfully within a diverse environment.

Health Disparities: What Pharmacy Students Need to Know

What is a *health disparity?* The first attempt at an official definition for *health disparities* was developed in September 1999, in response to a White House initiative. The National Institutes of Health (NIH), under the direction of then-director Dr. Harold Varmus, convened an NIH-wide working group, charged with developing a strategic plan for reducing health disparities. That group developed the first NIH definition of *health disparities*: "Health disparities are differences in the incidence, prevalence, mortality, and burden of diseases and other adverse health conditions that exist among specific population groups in the United States."[6]

In 2000, United States Public Law 106-525, also known as the Minority Health and Health Disparities Research and Education Act, which authorized the *National Center for Minority Health and Health Disparities*, provided a legal definition of health disparities: "A population is a health disparity population if there is a significant disparity in the overall rate of disease incidence, prevalence, morbidity, mortality or survival rates in the population as compared to the health status of the general population."[7] Recent studies and reports imply that there are differences not only in the services received by racial and ethnic minorities and people of lower socio-economic status, but also in the quality of those services.

The Office of Minority Health and Health Disparities (OMHD) has identified racial and ethnic minority populations as American Indian and Alaska Native, Asian, black or African American, Hispanic or Latino, and Native Hawaiian and Other Pacific Islander.[8] The OMHD further defines these populations as the following[8]:

- American Indian and Alaska native (AI/AN): people having origins in any of the original peoples of North and South America (including Central America), and who maintain tribal affiliation or community attachment

- Asian American: people having origins in any of the original peoples of the Far East, Southeast Asia, or the Indian subcontinent

- Black or African American: people having origins in any of the black racial groups of Africa

- Hispanic or Latino: people of Cuban, Mexican, Puerto Rican, South or Central American or other Spanish culture or origin, regardless of race

- Native Hawaiian and Other Pacific Islander (NHOPI): people having origins in any of the original peoples of Hawaii, Guam, Samoa, or other Pacific Islands

- Multiracial populations: people having origins in two or more of the federally designated racial categories

While death rates from breast cancer have declined during the 1990s, they remain higher among African American women. As reported in 2008 by the American Cancer Society, for African

American women the death rates were either flat or rising in 26 states in the U.S.[9] Women of racial and ethnic minorities are also less likely to receive Pap tests, which can detect precancerous changes in the cervix and could prevent cervical cancer. Death rates from cardiovascular diseases are about 30% higher among African Americans.

In March 2002, The Institute of Medicine (IOM) published its report, *Unequal Treatment: Confronting Racial and Ethnic Disparities in Healthcare.*[10] The IOM study committee found that health disparities exist in a number of areas including cardiovascular disease, HIV/AIDS, diabetes, cancer, mental illness and in routine treatments for common health problems. In 2004, the Sullivan Commission stated "The lack of minority health professionals is compounding the nation's persistent racial and ethnic health disparities. From cancer, heart disease, and HIV/AIDS to diabetes and mental health, African Americans, Hispanic Americans, and American Indians tend to receive less and lower quality healthcare than whites, resulting in higher mortality rates. The consequences of health disparities are grave and will only be remedied through sustained efforts and a national commitment."[11]

There are numerous factors that contribute to healthcare disparities. These include cultural and language barriers (e.g., the provider not understanding the health beliefs or health seeking behaviors of their patients) and the lack of interpretative services for patients with limited or lack of English proficiency. Other factors include the patients' inability to access care, utilize services, and navigate healthcare systems; economic factors (inability to pay, including lack of health insurance); locations where many minorities receive care (e.g., they are less likely to access care in a private physician's office); the cultural competency of the healthcare provider; and patients' general health literacy.

• Preceptor Pearls •

Unless you are thoroughly effective and fluent in conversational and medical terminology of the target language, always use qualified medical interpreters. This is especially important to ensure information is conveyed in a neutral and confidential manner. Speak slowly, not loudly, and look at the patient, not at the interpreter. Avoid interruptions. Do not use friends, family, or children for medical interpretation. Provide instructions in an organized format (e.g., a list) and have patients repeat their understanding of the message that was delivered. Return to an issue if you suspect it was not clear or may have been misunderstood.

In addition, there are factors identified by the IOM report that relate specifically to the patients' encounters with healthcare providers that may contribute to health disparities. These include the providers' real or perceived bias against minority patients, and stereotypes held by the providers about their patients' behaviors (e.g., response to pain) or health of a particular minority group (e.g., obesity). There is considerable empirical evidence that even well-intentioned non-Hispanic whites— who are not overtly biased and who do not believe that they are prejudiced—typically demonstrate unconscious implicit negative racial attitudes and stereotypes.[10]

For many racial and ethnic minorities in the U.S., good health is elusive and access to healthcare and prevention programs are often related to economic status, race or ethnicity, gender, education, disability, geographic location, or sexual orientation.[12] Some examples of health disparities in minorities cited by the CDC and the Indian Health Service (IHS) include the following:

- African Americans
  - Cancer. In 2001, the age-adjusted death rate for cancer was 25.4% higher for African Americans than for white Americans.[12]
  - Diabetes. African Americans born in the year 2000 face a two in five risk for diabetes. African Americans were more than twice as likely to have diabetes than white Americans. From 1980 through 2005, the age-adjusted prevalence of diagnosed diabetes doubled among African American males and increased 60% among African American females. However, of all groups observed, African American females had the highest overall prevalence of diabetes.[13]
  - Adult Immunization. In 2002, influenza vaccination coverage among adults 65 years of age and older was 70.2% for whites and 52% for African Americans.

- American Indians and Alaska Natives[14]
  - American Indians and Alaska Natives die at higher rates than other Americans from alcoholism (770%), tuberculosis (750%), diabetes (420%), accidents (280%), suicide (190%), and homicide (210%).[14]
  - The American Indian and Alaska Native people have long experienced lower health status when compared with other Americans. Lower life expectancy and the disproportionate disease burden exist perhaps because of inadequate education, disproportionate poverty, discrimination in the delivery of health services, and cultural differences. These are broad quality of life issues rooted in economic adversity and poor social conditions.

- Chronic diseases. Heart disease and cancer are the leading causes of death among American Indians and Alaska Natives. The prevalence of diabetes is more than twice that for all adults in the U.S., and the mortality rate from chronic liver disease is more than twice as high according to 2002 data.[12]

- Asian Americans
  - Access to healthcare. According to the 2000 U.S. census, Asian Americans represent 4.2% of the U.S. population. Overall, about 21% of Asian Americans lack health insurance compared to about 16% of the general population.
  - Asian Americans suffer disproportionately from certain types of cancer, tuberculosis, and Hepatitis B. The leading causes of death in the U.S. in 2001 for Asian Americans or Pacific Islanders were cancer, heart disease, stroke, unintentional injuries, diabetes, and chronic lower respiratory disease.[15]
  - Asian Americans have the highest rates of liver and stomach cancer for men and women and the third highest incidence rates of breast, lung, colon and rectal cancer for women.[15]

- Native Hawaiians and Other Pacific Islanders[12]
  - Native Hawaiians are 2.5 times more likely to be diagnosed with diabetes than non-Hispanic white residents of Hawaii of similar age.

- Native Hawaiians in Hawaii have almost twice the rate of asthma compared to other races in the state.
- In 2000, infant mortality among Native Hawaiians was 9.1 per 1,000, almost 60% higher than among whites.
- Asian Americans and Pacific islanders had the highest tuberculosis cases rates of any racial and ethnic population in 2001.

- Hispanics/Latinos
  - Hispanics are white, black, indigenous, Asian and every possible combination thereof, and originate from more than 20 countries. Hispanics are identified separately as an ethnicity; they can be of any race.[16]
  - Hispanics generally have lower mortality rates but higher morbidity rates compared with the overall U.S. population. As a result, morbidity and chronic disease management are areas of great concern for healthcare providers working with this population.[17]
  - There are differences in morbidity rates for chronic diseases within or among the Hispanic population as well. Among Hispanics, the diabetes death rate in 2000 was highest among Puerto Ricans, followed by rates for Mexican Americans and Cuban Americans.
  - Work related injuries. Mexican foreign-born workers accounted for 69% of the 2,440 fatally injured, foreign-born workers between 1995 and 2000.
  - In 2002, influenza vaccination coverage among adults 65 years of age and older was 70.2% for whites and 46.7% for Hispanics.
  - Hispanics born in the year 2000 face a two in five risk for diabetes; compared to whites, Hispanics are more than twice as likely to have diabetes.[13]

When a patient perceives the pharmacist as disinterested or less engaged in the patient-provider relationship, the patient is more likely to convey mistrust in you as the provider; he or she may not ask or respond to pertinent questions related to his or her care, refuse to accept treatment advice, and comply poorly with prescribed treatment. The pharmacist preceptor should educate students and make them aware that despite our best intentions, racial and ethnic disparities do exist in healthcare.

Access to Healthcare: Socioeconomic, Cultural, and Gender Issues

The fluctuating and difficult economic plight in the United States has resulted in an expanding healthcare crisis affecting all socioeconomic and cultural groups. Providers can cultivate a more astute and compassionate healthcare practice if they endeavor to comprehend the enlarging, similar, and different social and financial challenges encountered by residents of the U.S. needing and seeking healthcare. The federal and state governments have addressed these points in question through legislative changes promoting greater access to healthcare. However, these legislative changes have not sufficiently addressed the healthcare needs of the working poor and some middle-income workers. A growing number of workers are simultaneously struggling to meet daily living expenses and at the same time are overburdened with the financial obligations of paying for health insurance and/or chronic healthcare expenses. Healthcare providers can familiarize themselves with germane laws and public benefits, cultural issues, intervention strategies, as well as available resources to abate healthcare risk and contribute to more positive healthcare outcomes for their patients.

• Preceptor Pearls •

Direct patients to or provide them with information from pharmaceutical company patient assistance Internet sites, such as www.rxassist.org; www.rxhope.com; www.needymeds.com; www.rxoutreach.com; www.helpingpatients.org; www.Medicare.gov/prescriptions/home.asp; www.TogetherRxAccess.com; and www.ashp.org/PAP.

Access to Healthcare: A Socioeconomic Perspective

For many years the mounting healthcare crisis has been the focus of the U.S. federal government and a great concern to the American business community and workers. During the 1990s, the U.S. government under the Clinton Administration organized a national committee to develop a universal health insurance plan. This committee's proposals were not well-received by the insurance industry or by the medical community and failed to be voted into federal legislation. An important matter of interest was whether the government, healthcare providers, or the individual patients themselves would be making healthcare decisions under the proposed universal healthcare plan.

Later in the 1990s, the Personal Responsibility and Work Opportunity Reconciliation Act (PRWORA) of 1996 modified eligibility criteria for public (federal welfare) assistance programs. The law's cardinal intent was to limit cash assistance to, and dependency by, needy families by promoting job preparation and work and by supporting the formation and preservation of two-parent families. Additionally, with the PRWORA uninsured nonqualified aliens (nonimmigrant visitors and undocumented immigrants) are restricted to emergency Medicaid benefits and are left without health plan coverage for posthospital discharge care (i.e., outpatient medical care, home healthcare, inpatient rehabilitation, medical equipment and supplies, outpatient medications, and nursing home placement). Legal immigrants are currently ineligible for nonemergency Medicaid benefits for their first 5 years in the U.S., with some exceptions (Box 8.1).

Box 8.1 • Legal Immigrants Eligible for Nonemergency Medicaid Benefits

1. Refugees

2. Persons granted asylum and persons whose deportation is being withheld

3. Armed forces personnel or veterans and their dependent family members

4. Legal permanent residents with 40 Social Security qualifying quarters of work

5. Those receiving supplemental security income (SSI) benefits on August 22, 1996 and, subsequently, certified eligible under SSI as blind or disabled

The Balanced Budget Act of 1997 created the State Children's Health Insurance Plan (SCHIP). Under SCHIP each state offers health insurance for little or no cost for uninsured children up to the age of 19 years. State regulations for income eligibility and health services vary under each state-administered CHIP. SCHIP was intended to span the gap for children living in households that are income-ineligible for Medicaid benefits but who nonetheless reside in households with gross family incomes at or below twice the federal poverty level ($44,100 is twice the federal poverty level for a family of four in 2009).

During the latter part of the 1990s, health uninsurance was reduced for low income and some low moderate-income children with the expansion of the Medicaid Program and the initiation of healthcare benefits for children under the federally mandated SCHIP. In a few states, parents of low-income children were allowed to enroll in federal health programs. Subsequently, federal and state budget shortfalls in the past several years resulted in federal and state program cutbacks affecting eligibility for low-income adults and children and intensifying the healthcare crisis in the U.S.[18] While children's uninsurance rates remained steady the past several years, cutbacks in organized outreach efforts and more complex application processes have likely resulted in eligible children not becoming enrolled or losing eligibility.[19]

Beginning on January 1, 2006, Medicare drug discount cards began to be replaced by new Medicare Part D prescription plans. Medicare patients and their families can be directed to www.Medicare.gov for information on public and private programs that offer discounted or free medications, information on using generic medications and other means to reduce healthcare costs, and Medicare health plans that have prescription benefits.

The Family Medical Leave Act (FMLA) of 1993 provides workers of employers with 50 or more employees up to a total of 12 (nonconsecutive) work-weeks of unpaid leave during any rolling 12-month period for the following: (1) the birth and care of a newborn child; (2) the new adoption of a child by the employee; (3) the care of an immediate family member (spouse, child or parent) with a serious health condition, or (4) medical leave when the employee is unable to work because of a serious medical condition. Additionally, the National Defense Authorization Act of 2008 amends the FMLA of 1993 to allow a "spouse, son, daughter, parent or next of kin" to have up to 26 workweeks of leave to care for a "member of the Armed Forces, including a member of the National Guard or Reserves, who is undergoing medical treatment, recuperation, or therapy, is otherwise in outpatient status, or is otherwise on the temporary disability retired list, for a serious injury or illness." For serious medical conditions, the employee using FMLA may be required to obtain medical forms from the ill family member's physician annually or as frequently as monthly. Some employers have bureaucratic procedures that make access to FMLA benefits difficult to obtain. Employees with available paid leave may be able to use vacation time and/or sick time to care for themselves or their family member. However, serious health conditions frequently result in employees taking unpaid medical leave, compromising already strained family finances.

In the U.S., most of the elderly have health insurance coverage through Medicare. In 2006, 46.5 million nonelderly Americans were without health insurance due to public program limits and decreasing health insurance coverage by employees. Over 2 million more individuals became uninsured between 2005 and 2006 with 18% nonelderly in 2006 having no health plan coverage. Although enrollment in Medicaid and SCHIP increased health insurance coverage for low income children, the number of adult uninsured increased. Adults without children usually do not qualify for

Medicaid unless they are severely disabled. Working families account for more than four out of five (82%) of the uninsured; of these, 71% reside in households with at least one full-time worker and 11% are in households with a part-time worker. Uninsured adults over the age of 30 years represent 61% of uninsured adults. U.S. citizens account for almost 80% of the uninsured.[20]

There are more than 9 million parents who are uninsured. About 80% of uninsured individuals are adults, and 17% to 19% are children (most low income children have Medicaid or CHIP).[21] Working adults with gross family incomes at or below twice the federal poverty level represent two in five uninsured Americans. In the economic downturns of recent years, employers have increasingly decided to stop offering healthcare benefits to their employees or are offering plans that are less generous and inclusive.[22] At least two-thirds of nonelderly uninsured adults are employed; they work for employers that do not offer health plan coverage or they cannot afford the coverage that is offered to them. In 2005 60% of employers offered health insurance compared to 69% who offered health insurance in 2000. Adults and racial and ethnic minorities represent a disproportionate number of the uninsured. About one-half of the uninsured individuals are (non-Hispanic) white and about one-half are ethnic and racial minorities.[21]

Most uninsured low-income adults work at jobs that offer no heath plan or cannot afford to participate in the high-cost health plan offered.[22] Working people and their families who don't have employer-sponsored health plans represent an annual $45 billion expenditure per year ($33 billion in Medicaid and SCHIP and $12 in uncompensated care costs; this amount totaled $31 billion in 1999). One-third of low-paid workers do not have health insurance; this represents a 9% increase since 1996. A lot of public money goes to pay for healthcare for individuals who are working and that amount of money goes up every year.[23]

Between the years 2000 and 2003, the number of uninsured adults grew by an additional 5 million. Increased uninsurance has affected low-moderate- and high-income workers but mostly low-income young workers. The ranks of low-income adults have increased with the shift of some middle-income adults to low-income status. Sixty-nine percent of employers offered health benefits in 2000 compared to 60% in 2007. The offer rate is 45% in 2007 compared to 57% in 2000 for firms with three to nine workers. Among firms with 200 or more employees the offer rate is 98% to 99%, a rate that has remained consistent.[24] It is anticipated that the rate of uninsured individuals will continue to increase with the trend of declining employer-sponsored health coverage.[18] Also, employers who maintain health coverage for their employees are incrementally increasing employee cost-sharing (i.e., increasing premiums, copays, coinsurance and costs of spousal and family coverage; thinning benefits, etc.).[25]

Eighty-three percent of noncitizen immigrants are in working families; they are similarly likely as citizens to have at least one full-time worker in the family. Noncitizens generally are employed in low wage labor or service jobs that do not offer health plan benefits. Immigrants represent 13% of the total U.S. population, and 69% of those are in the U.S. legally. Because noncitizens represent a small share of the U.S. population, noncitizens are not the primary reason for the nation's growing uninsured problem, as citizens make up the majority of the uninsured. Noncitizens also receive substantially less healthcare than citizens for both primary and preventative care. Additionally, noncitizens are considerably less likely to go to an emergency room compared to citizens.[26]

Racial and ethnic minorities in the U.S. have incomes and rates of health insurance coverage that are disproportionately low compared with their white counterparts. Low-income Hispanics, although more likely to have a stable (full-time) income across several years compared to other low-income groups, have the highest uninsured rates.[18] Thirty-seven percent of nonelderly Hispanics are uninsured (87% of the uninsured Hispanics are in working families) compared to 14% for whites. Sixty percent of Hispanics reside in households below twice the federal poverty level compared to 23% of whites.[27]

Public policy (lack of increased funding for several years for the IHS) has contributed to poor health, shorter life expectancies, and the frequency of disease for American Indians and Alaska Natives. Many Medicaid-eligible, low-income American Indians are not enrolled in Medicaid.[28] Fifty-six percent of American Indians do not have access to the IHS because they live in urban areas and have to travel to their home reservation to receive their IHS care, or because they belong to a nonfederally recognized tribe and nearly half have incomes below twice the federal poverty level.[29,30]

Eight in 10 African Americans reside in working families, but 23% are uninsured, 21% receive Medicaid benefits, and about half have family incomes below twice the federal poverty level. Their uninsured rates are about one and one-half times that of whites. The welfare reform of the 1990s transitioned many individuals into low-paying jobs with no or unaffordable health benefits. Transitional Medicaid benefits have been denied to families moving from public welfare programs to the workforce due to insufficient program administration and outreach efforts.[30]

Asian American and Pacific Islanders represent a number of widely diverse subgroups. For example, Korean Americans have 48% job-based health coverage while Japanese Americans have 77% coverage. These sub-groups have different rates of self-employment and of work in small businesses (which are less likely to offer health benefits and are an important factor in uninsurance rates), citizenship, refugee status, income status, and participation in Medicaid despite rates of poverty that are higher than for the white U.S. population.[31]

Women and Access to Healthcare

Compared to men, women are less likely to have employer-sponsored health insurance and more probable to have dependent coverage. Uninsured women account for 18% of the nonelderly population of women. These uninsured women characteristically are unable to qualify for Medicaid or employer-sponsored plans and cannot meet the expenses of individual policies. Over 17 million women are uninsured. Nearly eight out of 10 (79%) uninsured women are in families with at least one part-time or full-time worker. Almost two-thirds (65%) of uninsured women are in families with at least one adult working full-time. Just 21% of uninsured women are in families without workers.[32]

Compared to non-Hispanic white women, Latinas and African-American women are more probable to have a low income and less likely to have job-related health insurance coverage. More than one-third of Latinas are uninsured (37%), which is more than twice as likely as white women (16%). Twenty percent of African-American women are uninsured. The higher rates of uninsurance for women of color are related to lower rates of job-based coverage. Latinas and African American women have disparities in access to healthcare because of health status, uninsurance rates, access to doctors, ability to pay healthcare expenses, availability of transportation and childcare, utilization of preventative services, and perceptions and satisfaction with quality. Latinas relate that language barriers make communication with healthcare providers complex while African American women experience an increasing hardship of preventable illness.[33]

Part-time employment and breaks in employment leave low-income families without coverage or with gaps in healthcare coverage. The Consolidated Omnibus Budget Reconciliation Act (COBRA) of 1986 allows some employees and their families who lose their health plan benefits due to specified circumstances (e.g., voluntary or involuntary job loss, reduction in work hours, changes in jobs, death, divorce, and other life events) the right to continue group health coverage under the former employer's group health plan for limited periods of time. The cost is 102% of the entire premium (total of employer and employee expenses) and applies to group health plans sponsored by employers with 20 or more employees. However, the cost of COBRA benefits is cost-prohibitive for low- and moderate-income families already struggling to pay for basic family necessities due to job loss, underemployment, or part-time employment.

The Commonwealth Fund Biennial Health Insurance Survey revealed that gaps in health insurance coverage and large medical bills reduced individuals' ability to access appropriate healthcare.[18] About 20 million American families experienced problems in 2003 with paying medical bills; about one-third of these families were uninsured, and about two-thirds had health insurance. The presence of health coverage does not protect people from high out-of-pocket medical costs, and nearly half of all personal bankruptcies are due in part to medical expenses. Additionally, due to the economic recessions of recent years, some state Medicaid programs have reduced benefits, imposed limits (i.e., monthly prescription limits), or imposed copays. About one-half of all families with medical bill problems are low-income. Almost two-thirds of all families with medical bill problems also reported difficulty with paying for basic family necessities (shelter, food, or transportation) due to medical debts.[34]

In 2003, 12.3 million working-age people (3 million uninsured) with chronic health conditions resided in families having problems in paying medical bills, making them more likely to delay or skip necessary medical care. Also in 2003, approximately one in five persons' healthcare expenses were in excess of 10% of family income.[35] In 2004, individuals with healthcare expenses paid on average 34% of their total healthcare costs.[36] Chronic conditions usually call for regular medical follow-up and higher out-of-pocket medical costs. Of the 3 million uninsured, 42% went without necessary care, 65% delayed care, and 71% went without needed prescriptions. Of the 12.3 million working-age people, 64% were contacted by a collection agency and 50% had to borrow funds. Recent studies have discovered that doubling of a copay from $10 to $20 resulted in significant cutbacks in the use of important prescription medications (i.e., diabetes and high cholesterol).[37]

Individuals with chronic health problems are frequently dependent on others for basic needs such as psychological support and medical transportation, and in more complicated medical situations, for help with activities of daily living (bathing, dressing, mobility, and/or feeding). The frequency of medical appointments for the chronically ill person can result in lost income for the family member who must give up work hours or employment to care or provide support for the ill individual. When the adult providing support is the single or primary wage earner in the household, the combination of lost income and emotional stress of caring for the chronically ill person exacerbate family psychosocial stressors. If the adult providing support works for a small employer, there is an increased risk for job loss due to the employer being unable to accommodate the employee's work tardiness or absences.[38]

The Healthcare Provider Role: A Bridge to Making Healthcare Accessible

It is important to consider that despite the differences between ethnic, age, and cultural groups noted above, people have many things in common. Also, an advantage of diversity and differences between individuals is that we can learn from our patients. Healthcare providers can improve access to healthcare and reduce health risk for their patients with even small but important endeavors such as providing warm, friendly greetings, as well as visual observation and active listening to perceive commonalities and health concerns. Health literacy assessments assist providers to understand how individuals learn about and adapt to their health problems and treatment plan. Consumer confidence and trust are promoted by the presentation of treatment matters of concern in a way that develops common healthcare goals. It is important to identify what patients hope to accomplish by jointly planning for treatment. Helping patients to understand and prioritize their treatment plan and healthcare strategies and to comprehend how healthcare outcomes will be measured is integral to collaborative patient-provider healthcare.

Strategies for Improving Healthcare Services

A strategy for improving the delivery of healthcare services is for preceptors and students to gain knowledge about the healthcare views, ideals, and cultural communication styles of different ethnic groups (Box 8.2) Another essential approach is to take time to appreciate the individual's identity, literacy level, and degree of acculturation/assimilation (Box 8.3). The student's ability to assess the patient and family's abilities to comprehend and accommodate to their disease management process is integral to understanding health literacy, health education, and compliance issues (Box 8.4). Finally, ascertaining and enhancing the patient and family's knowledge and use of available resources provides the patient with an indispensable support system for successful self-management of his/her disease or acute or chronic condition (Box 8.5).

Box 8.2 • Objective: To Gain Knowledge About Healthcare Beliefs, Values, and Cultural Communication Styles of Different Ethnic Groups

Strategies:

1. Learn about attitudes regarding frankness about health problems (e.g., is it acceptable to speak to the patient or the family about prognosis, death and dying?).

2. Learn who is the decision-maker or head of the household in your patient's culture.

3. Determine whether the patient or family adheres to traditional non-American cultural practices or the American model (i.e., the patient or legal representative is responsible for healthcare decisions) of decision-making in healthcare.

4. Determine whether there are any characteristic or culture-specific meanings to particular health conditions and diseases.

5. Consider the cultural norms regarding social distance, eye contact, communication, and physical contact between the genders or between the patient and healthcare provider.

6. Determine whether healthcare decisions are individual-centered or family-centered.

Box 8.3 • Objective: To Appreciate the Individual's Identity, Literacy Level, and Degree of Acculturation/Assimilation

Strategies:

1. Evaluate own assumptions about who is a "good patient."

2. Assume mutual respect.

3. Greet patients and their families with a warm smile and steady handshake (when culturally appropriate).

4. Make physical contact (e.g., handshake, hand on the shoulder of an elderly person, pat on the head of a small child, etc.) with the very young, elderly, or infirm family members.

5. Ask where the patient and the family were born and how long they have been in the United States.

6. Inquire about the languages he/she speaks and ask which language is the one he/she is most comfortable in talking and receiving written information.

7. Ask the patient and/or family what concerns them most about the illness/disease.

8. Observe the patient or parent's ability to complete consent and intake forms to screen for potential learning and literacy issues.

Box 8.4 • Objective: Assessment of the Patient and Family's Abilities to Comprehend and Adapt to the Disease (integral to understanding health literacy, health education and compliance issues)

Strategies:

1. Promote patient confidence.

2. Understand that an authoritarian posture decreases patient empowerment and participation and may increase dependency on the provider.

3. Ask about the patient's support system (e.g., who is available to provide financial support, emotional support, medical transportation, physical care, care of other family members, etc.).

4. Use social persuasion (family support).

5. Acknowledge that the patient or family may already be involved in healthcare self-management.

6. Reinterpret symptoms and recommendations as necessary.

7. Provide regular (re)assessment of progress and issues as well as goal-setting and problem-solving support.

8. Support the patient or family with setting specific, attainable healthcare goals.

9. Negotiate during healthcare encounters.

Box 8.5 • Objective: Ascertain and Expand the Patient and Family's Knowledge and Use of Available Resources to Provide the Patient with an Integral Support

System for Successful Self-Management and Self-Efficacy

Strategies:

1. View patient encounters as opportunities for information-sharing and as a partnership with the patients and their families.

2. Assist with weighing the costs and advantages of the treatment options.

3. Because language barriers are sometimes misinterpreted as noncompliance, obtain competent, nonbiased interpretive services to increase patient participation and satisfaction, as well as confidence, compliance, and positive outcomes.

4. Provide patient with information about Medicaid and CHIP, governmental programs that assist poor and low-income children and/or adults with healthcare expenses that are accessed through state agencies.

5. Take advantage of the on-site interpretive services that Medicaid managed care health plan member services departments can assist with providing.

6. Inform patients that Medicaid benefits include medical transportation services to medical appointments and to pick up prescription medications.

7. Direct patients to or provide them with information from drug company patient assistance Internet sites, such as www.rxassist.org; www.rxhope.com; www.needymeds.com; www.rxoutreach.com; www.helpingpatients.org; www.Medicare.gov/prescriptions/home.asp; www.TogetherRxAccess.com; and www.ashp.org/PAP/.

8. Direct patients to www.Medicare.gov for assistance with Medicare information on public and private programs that offer discounted or free medication, information on using generic medications and other means to reduce healthcare costs, and Medicare health plans that have prescription benefits.

9. Inform patients that workers can obtain employer-specific or Department of Labor forms to request Family Medical Leave Act (FMLA) benefits from their human resources office.

10. Remind patients that workers may be eligible for short-term and/or long-term disability and/or COBRA benefits through their employer's human resources office.

11. Inform patients that individuals with terminal illness or severe disability expected to last 12 months or more may be eligible for Social Security Disability Income (SSDI) (may eventually receive Medicare benefits with this) or Supplemental Security Income (SSI) and Medicaid benefits from the Social Security Administration (1-800-772-1213 or www.ssa.gov/disability/).

12. Inform patients that consumers with outstanding hospital bills may be eligible for hospital charity care or indigent care programs.

Box 8.5 • Objective: Ascertain and Expand the Patient and Family's Knowledge and Use of Available Resources to Provide the Patient with an Integral Support (cont'd)

13. Provide patients with information about Consumer Credit Counseling Services (1-800-493-2222 or 1-800-388-2227, or www.moneymanagement.org), an agency that helps consumers negotiate reasonable payment arrangements.

14. Inform patients that the state insurance commissioner's office may be able to provide information about high-risk insurance pools.

15. Inform patients that local or state-wide hospital districts may be able to provide free or discounted healthcare services.

16. Provide patients with information about the Special Supplemental Nutrition Program for Women, Infants, and Children (known more commonly as the WIC Program), which provides services to low-income infants, children up to the age of 5 years, and pregnant women. WIC services include nutritional supplements and free or very low-cost immunizations.

17. Inform patients that city and county health departments/clinics provide free or very low-cost immunizations and other healthcare services.

The Importance of Health Literacy in Healthcare Outcomes

What is health literacy? *Healthy People 2010* defines health literacy as the degree to which individuals have the capacity to obtain, process, and understand basic health information and services needed to make appropriate health decisions.[39] More simply stated, it is the patient's ability to read, understand, and act on healthcare information.

People with low health literacy are less likely to understand written and verbal information or instructions given to them by physicians, pharmacists, nurses, or insurance companies. They are frequently unable to follow directions such as those found on medication labels or appointment schedules.[39] Persons with the most health problems and the greatest need for self-management skills often have the poorest health literacy skills.[39]

Healthcare systems as we know them today have created an incredible challenge for persons with low health literacy skills. Healthcare providers and others rely heavily on the use of the written word to communicate. Directions on consent forms, instructions for surgery or procedures and medication directions can be complex making it difficult for persons with low health literacy skills. There is only one medication frequency instruction, "take one tablet daily," that is understood greater than 90% of the time. The direction "take one tablet twice a day" is understood less frequently. HIV positive adults with low functional health literacy miss more treatment doses than patients with high health literacy because they do not understand instructions on how to take their medications.[40] Research has shown that health literacy is a stronger predictor of health status than age, income, employment status, education level, or racial or ethnic makeup of the individual.

• Preceptor Pearls •

Assess a patient's understanding by asking open-ended questions. Do not say "Do you understand?" Be alert to nonverbal clues that may help assess a patient's understanding of the information provided.

According to the National Adult Literacy Survey (NALS), the 2003 NAAL assessment questions were developed to be able to measure three types of literacy[41]:

- Prose literacy. The ability to search, understand and use continuous texts (e.g., brochures, education materials, and news stories).

- Document literacy. The ability to search, understand and use noncontinuous tasks (e.g., medication label, job application, map, bus schedule).

- Quantitative literacy. The ability to identify and perform computations, either alone or sequentially using numbers embedded in printed materials, (e.g., completing an order form or balancing a check book).

Examples of survey questions included the following:

- Find the list of stores that sell milk in the yellow pages.

- Read a sign-out sheet to determine if a person has returned.

- Write in and subtract a $53 check on a check ledger

- Fill in name, address, and phone number on an order form.

- Describe what the point or gist of this article is about.

- Calculate the cost of a certain lunch.

- List facts stated in the article.

- Find information about disability.

The Impact of Low Health Literacy

The 1992 NALS indicated that 75% of Americans who reported having a chronic illness (>6 months) had limited literacy.[42] The survey estimated that as many as 44 million people in the U.S. cannot read a prescription label, read a bus schedule, or interpret directions on a map. In addition, 53 million more are marginally literate. The average American reads between the 8th and 9th grade levels. The NALS survey also illustrated that adults in America with low literacy are comprised of 41% English-speaking whites, 22% English-speaking African Americans, 22% Spanish-speaking Americans, and 15% other. Practitioners who have worked with low-literacy patients for years are often surprised at the poor reading skills of some of their most poised and articulate patients.[43]

Some key findings of the 2003 NAAL indicate that the percentage of adults with below basic document literacy decreased 2% between 1992 and 2003 and the percentage of adults with below basic quantitative literacy decreased by 4%.[44] The percentage of adults with basic literacy did not change significantly between 1992 and 2003. Field interviewers determined that 2% of adults in 2003 and 3% in 1992 could not be tested because they spoke a language other than English or Spanish and were unable to communicate in English or Spanish. It is highly encouraged that both preceptors and students review the report *National Assessment of Adult Literacy (NAAL): A First Look at the Literacy of America's Adults in the 21ˢᵗ Century*.[44] Figures 8.1 through 8.3 compare the results of the 1992 and 2003 surveys. Recognizing the literacy limitations of our patients can help us identify tools to better educate them about the use of their medications.

Inadequate health literacy increases with age. Patients with low literacy skills frequently utilize emergency rooms or primary care facilities and community-based health centers for primary care services. Because they are unlikely to obtain preventive health services, patients with low literacy make more unnecessary follow-up visits, are more likely to be hospitalized, and are more susceptible to medical errors.[45]

Patients with poor health literacy are more likely to have a chronic disease and less likely to understand their condition and obtain the healthcare they need. Only 50% of low literate patients know the symptoms of hypoglycemia or the definition of a normal blood sugar. Sixty percent of low literate patients do not know that exercise could lower their blood pressure.[46] Low literate patients

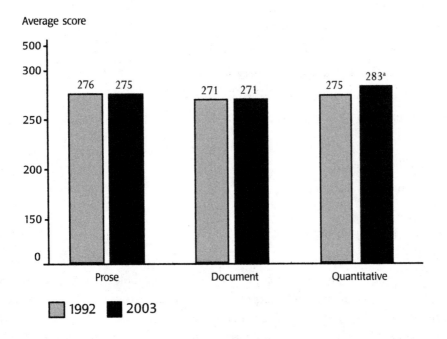

Figure 8.1. Average prose, document, and quantitative literacy scores of adults: 1992 and 2003 average scores. There was no significant change in prose and document literacy between 1992 and 2003, and an increase in quantitative literacy.

[a]Significantly different from 1992.

Note: Adults are defined as people 16 years of age and older living in households or prisons. Adults who could not be interviewed due to language spoken or cognitive or mental disabilities (3% in 2003 and 4% in 1992) are excluded from this figure.

Source: U.S. Department of Education, Institute of Education Sciences, National Center for Education Statistics, 1992 National Adult Literacy Survey and 2003 National Assessment of Adult Literacy.

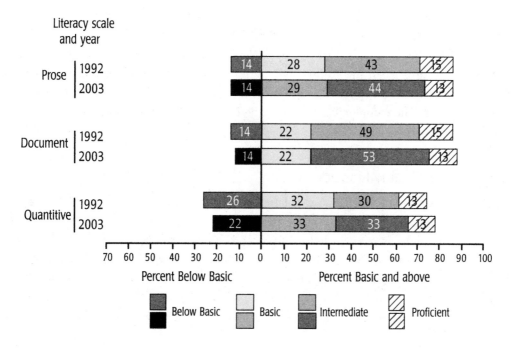

Figure 8.2. Percentage of adults in each prose, document, and quantitative literacy level: 1992 and 2003.

[a]Significantly different from 1992.

Note: Detail may not sum to totals because of rounding. Adults are defined as people 16 years of age and older living in households or prisons. Adults who could not be interviewed due to language spoken or cognitive or mental disabilities (3% in 2003 and 4% in 1992) are excluded from this figure.

Source: U.S. Department of Education, Institute of Education Sciences, National Center for Education Statistics, 1992 National Adult Literacy Survey and 2003 National Assessment of Adult Literacy.

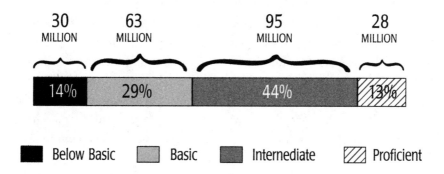

Figure 8.3. Number of adults in each prose literacy level. Prose literacy levels are below basic and demonstrates no more than the most *simple* and *concrete* literacy skills. Basic—can perform simple and everyday literacy activities; intermediate—can perform moderately challenging literacy activities; and proficient—can perform complex and challenging literacy activities.

with asthma are less likely to know how to use an inhaler. Low literate mothers are less likely to know how to read a thermometer.

Nonadherence to prescribed medication therapy is a common problem especially for patients with chronic diseases because patients with low health literacy skills often have limited knowledge of their medical condition. The complexity of dosage frequency or medication administration can lead to poor medication adherence.[46]

Assessing Patient Health Literacy

Because pharmacists are usually readily accessible to most patients or consumers, they may often be in a position to be the first healthcare provider to recognize that a patient is having health literacy problems. Some of the more important skills that preceptors should teach their students are methods to assess their patient's functional health literacy.[47] In addition, students should learn to be alert for "red flags" that can identify problems in this area. For example, a patient may say, "I forgot my glasses. Can you read the directions on the label to me?" or "I'll read this when I get home." Patients may make excuses, joke or use humor, become quiet or passive, or pretend they can read.

Effective Communication to Enhance Health Literacy

The use of "brown bag" or medication reviews with patients can be helpful ways to identify and address problems with health literacy. Teach students to ask open-ended questions to assess if a patient is able to name his/her medications or explain why and when medications should be taken. Use this discussion to identify areas of confusion and to answer patients' questions. Knowing how frequently patients are refilling their medication can also provide a clue about their medication adherence. Be alert to patients who have difficulty expressing medical concerns or has no questions. Do not ask, "Do you understand?" Create an environment where patients are not embarrassed to ask you questions or express their concerns. Patients should feel comfortable in indicating to you that they do not understand the information you may be trying to convey. Speak clearly and use plain language; avoid medical jargon to explain medical information.

The most successful interventions for promoting medication adherence include the use of both written and verbal communication. Often using visual tools or pictures helps the patients understand the action or behavior that is being recommended. Students should be taught to choose words that are at the 6th grade level and that show respect for a patient's culture. For example, if you are working with a patient to try and reduce fat intake, introduce the subject by saying to "cut back" rather than to "eliminate" or "replace" lard with vegetable oil. Many patients do not understand what it means to take a medication on an empty stomach or twice or three times a day. The communication should emphasize the desired behavior rather than medical or medication facts. Using the "teach-back" or "show me" methods with all patients are still reliable methods to determine the extent of patients' understanding the instructions for taking their medication.[43]

Be a role model to your students and show them patient-centered communication skills. Teach them to engage in a conversation with patients; do not dictate to patients. Demonstrate to students how to encourage patients to ask questions. Speak slowly and start with the most important information or message first. Use repetition and demonstrate when follow-up phone calls may be helpful. Teach them, when appropriate, to give instructions not only to patients, but also to family members or other caregivers. Most importantly, teach students to listen actively to their patients, to learn about, and to address their patients' concerns.

Teach students to print out directions or label medications with the time indicated to give patients clear directions to follow. For example, for twice-a-day directions you may indicate to take at 9 a.m. and 5 p.m., or 8 a.m. and 6 p.m. Tailor the medication schedule to fit a patient's daily routine. The use of colors as codes or the use of pictures such as the sun and/or the moon can be used to indicate morning and night. Likewise, the use of charts, calendars, and picture books may also be helpful.

When preparing written materials to give to patients make sure that the documents are easy to read; write information at a 5th or 6th grade reading level. For most of the population anything above an 8th grade level, especially if dealing with medical information or terms, may be too difficult. Make the document or information look easy to read. Use bullet points and short sentences, and have lots of white space on the document or leaflet. Remember, for elderly patients you want to print or use a larger font for any written material that you give to them. Keep a patient's culture in mind when developing written information for patients. For example, in some cultures a patient many respond or adhere to prescribed therapy if you say something is "important" rather than "helpful." If the patient is having difficulty understanding written or verbal directions, a good approach may be to say, "Many people have trouble reading and remembering these instructions. How can I help you?"

Students should learn to deliver short, concise messages. Patients usually remember less than 50% of the information provided during each encounter. Teach students to use common, everyday language when speaking to their patients. Some common examples[43]:

- "For pain" or "pain killer" instead of "analgesic"
- "Make bones weaker" instead of "osteoporosis"
- "By mouth" instead of "oral"
- "Swelling" instead of "edema"
- "Sore or painful joints instead" of "osteoarthritis"
- "Treat cancer" instead of "chemotherapy"
- "High blood pressure" instead of "hypertension"

Students should know when and how to use an interpreter. Many healthcare providers rely on family members and coworkers to serve as interpreters. Use a skilled interpreter, one who is competent to interpret and translate medically related issues. Coworkers or staff may overestimate their own skills and abilities, especially when a patient wishes to expand the discussion or requests additional information. Even patients who are bilingual may choose to communicate in their first language when the issues are emotional or involve their health. Remember to teach students how to look for nonverbal cues that a communication problem exists.

• Preceptor Pearls •

When talking to patients whose primary language is not English, speak clearly and slowly using a caring tone of voice. When possible, use pictures to help patients understand; repeat message if necessary to assure understanding.

In summary, a person with good health literacy skills should be able to do the following:

- Understand diagnosis or condition.
- Understand medication instructions (e.g., take on an empty stomach, what twice a day means, etc.).
- Repeat back healthcare information and demonstrate the ability to utilize tools to manage chronic conditions such as a glucometer.
- Understand consent forms and accurately complete standard screening forms.
- Initiate questions with health providers.
- Understand how to effectively use insurance.

Both preceptors and students must demonstrate good communication skills including empathy, listening, and appreciative inquiry. The first impression you make on your patients can make a big difference. Demonstrate an attitude of helpfulness, caring, and respect, and put patients at ease so that they feel comfortable in asking questions

Cultural Competency in Modern Healthcare

The National Center for Cultural Competence (NCCC) defines culture as an integrated pattern of human behavior that includes thoughts, communication, languages, beliefs, practices, customs, courtesies, rituals, manners of interacting, roles, relationships, and expected behaviors of a racial, ethnic, religious, social, or political group.[48] The NCCC states that there are numerous reasons to justify the need for cultural competence in healthcare at the patient-provider level.[49] These include but are not limited to the following:

- The perception of illness and disease and their causes varies by culture.
- Diverse belief systems exist related to health, healing, and wellness.
- Culture influences health-seeking behaviors and attitudes toward healthcare providers.
- Individual preferences affect traditional and nontraditional approaches to healthcare.
- Patients must overcome personal experiences of biases within healthcare systems.
- Health providers from culturally and linguistically diverse groups are underrepresented in the current service delivery system.

Assessing Cultural Competency

The U.S. Department of Health and Human Services (HHS) Office of Minority Health defines cultural competency as the ability of the healthcare providers and organizations to understand, respect, and respond effectively to the cultural and linguistic needs brought by patients to the healthcare setting. Pharmacy students must learn how to communicate with and provide direct patient care services to patients of varying cultures and healthcare preferences. Students and preceptors should be able to demonstrate understanding and respect for patients with differing health beliefs and health seeking behaviors and practices, thereby demonstrating cultural proficiency. Preceptors and students must appreciate their patients' cultural beliefs; this is critical in the delivery of optimal care.

• Preceptor Pearls •

How a patient expresses pain can vary significantly between cultures as well as between men and women. In some cultures stoicism is expected.

Asian Americans represent a wide variety of languages, dialects, and cultures. They are as different from one another as individuals from non-Asian cultures. According to the 2000 census, Asians and Pacific Islanders are comprised of the following: 25.4% Chinese, 19.3% Filipino, 17.6% Asian Indian, 11.7% Vietnamese, 8.3% Japanese, and 4.2% Pacific Islander.[50] More than half (54%) of the Asian and Pacific Islander population live in the West, 17% live in the South, 18% in the Northeast, and 11% in the Midwest. Nearly 40% of Asian Americans residing in the U.S. live in California. The greatest percentages of Asians are in Honolulu, San Francisco, San Jose, San Diego, Seattle, and Los Angeles. Language is the most prominent barrier for Asians and Pacific Islanders. According to the 2000 census, 66% of Asians and Pacific Islanders speak a language other than English at home. About 38% of Asian Americans do not speak English fluently.[50]

Although Cuban Americans are often classified as Hispanics or Latinos, their customs and traditions differ from Mexican American, Central American, or South American. Latinos/Hispanics come from different nations and cultures. According to the 2000 census, Latinos are classified as follows: 58.5% Mexican American, 9.6% Puerto Rican, 4.8% Central American, 3.8% South American, 3.5% Cuban American, and 19.8% other Latino/Hispanic. The largest concentration is in four cities: New York, Los Angeles, Chicago, and San Antonio.[51] Data from the Kaiser study indicates that about 60% of Hispanic adults speak Spanish at home, 20% are bilingual, and 20% are English dominant.[51] Kaiser data also indicates that Hispanics are the most likely to be uninsured. This is because the jobs held by many Hispanics do not provide health benefits (e.g., migrant workers, day laborers, housekeepers, etc.).

The national standards for culturally and linguistically appropriate services (CLAS) in healthcare were set forth by the U.S. Department of Health and Human Services Office of Minority Health in order to provide guidelines on policies and practices aimed at developing culturally appropriate systems of care.[52] The scope of these standards, the teaching approaches, and the challenges to consider when implementing these standards are applicable to all health professionals.

Cultural competence has evolved from the making of assumptions about patients on the basis of their background to the implementation of the principles of patient-centered care, including exploration, empathy, and responsiveness to patients' needs values and preferences.[1] It is important not to stereotype patients broadly based on their ethnicity or culture. Unfortunately, this frequently happens when our care is based on textbook methods of addressing patients within the same cultural population such as Hispanics, Asians, or African Americans. There is no one way to treat any racial or ethnic group.

• Preceptor Pearls •

To perform a cultural assessment, identify or assess the following:

- The patient's level of ethnic identity (e.g., first versus third generation)

- Language or communication barriers

- Influence of religion, spiritual beliefs, or supernatural effects on the patient's health belief system

- Concerns about racial or ethnic discrimination or bias

- Educational and literacy, including health literacy levels

- Current economic status

- Cultural health beliefs and practices

- Influence of family in compliance to prescribed treatment plan

- Influence of family in the medical decision-making process

There are many aspects relating to cultural competence that preceptors need to teach their students. These include fundamental knowledge such as concepts of race, culture, ethnicity, family structure, gender roles, religion, death, differing communication styles, and principals of disease management as they relate to certain cultures. Preceptors can demonstrate and teach effective communication skills, relationship building, language proficiency or effective use of interpreters, ability to differentiate varying views of illness and healing, and how to recognize culture related problems. Preceptors can teach students how to integrate the patients' beliefs into the overall treatment strategy or plan.

Lastly, complementary and alternative medicine (CAM) has growing social, economic, and clinical significance in the U.S. It is important for pharmacist preceptors and students to understand the implications of CAM for their patients: what it is, who uses it, and why.

• Preceptor Pearls •

Ask patients if they are taking any home remedies (herbs, teas, etc.) or if they have sought advice for their condition from others including family, friends, or alternative healers (e.g., abuela, sobrador, or curandero).

The National Center for Complementary and Alternative Medicine (NCCAM) defines CAM as a broad range of healing philosophies (schools of thought), approaches, and therapies that mainstream Western (conventional) medicine does not commonly use, accept, study, understand, or make available.[53] A few of the many CAM practices include the use of acupuncture, herbs, homeopathy, therapeutic massage, and traditional oriental medicine to promote well-being or treat health conditions. Many CAM therapies are called *holistic*, which generally means they consider the whole person, including physical, mental, and spiritual aspects.[54]

Cultural Competence: A Continuing Learning Process

One of the most important traits that a preceptor can model for students is respect and understanding of their patients. Addressing your patient with the appropriate salutation or title can be extremely important and effective when communicating with patients with diverse backgrounds. For example, in Mexico and throughout Latin America, a licensed professional such as an accountant or administrator, is addressed as "licensciado." Professionals with a doctoral degree in any field, medical or nonmedical, are addressed as "doctor." Although many assimilate to the mainstream culture in the United States, many Latin Americans tend to retain their language and cultural identity. Simple gestures such as using the appropriate salutation (e.g., Mr., Mrs., Señor, Señora, etc.), asking permission before touching the patient (e.g., to take a blood pressure), honoring elders, and demonstrating respect for patients' culture can go a long way in establishing a positive patient-provider relationship. Learn how to demonstrate respect in various cultural contexts.

• Preceptor Pearls •

- Ask patients what language they prefer when discussing their medical care and in what language they prefer to receive any written healthcare information.

- When first interacting with patients who were born in another country, it is best to use their last name when addressing them.

- Do not be insulted if a patient does not look at you directly in the eye or fails to ask questions. In many cultures it is not respectful to look at another person, especially someone in authority or highly respected like a healthcare provider.

The following example illustrates some of the challenges that pharmacists and students may encounter in dealing with ethnically and culturally diverse patients. An elderly Iranian woman has been admitted to the hospital where you work. Neither the patient nor her family reads, speaks, or understands English. Her Muslim faith requires modesty, and she may not be the primary decision maker in her healthcare. Using this example, how would you teach students to interact with this patient and/or her family? You might use one or more of the following services appropriate for this patient: the use of interpreter staff; written information materials and consent forms that have been translated to Farsi; appropriate food choices; and clinical and support staff who understands how to interact appropriately with the patient and family.

Consider this example as well: an elderly African American patient's blood pressure has been difficult to control since the doctor changed his therapy to a new medication. If you teach your students how to assess the patient through a thoughtful and respectful inquiry, they may discover that a distant relative of the patient had been involved with the Tuskegee Syphilis Study. For many African Americans, the Tuskegee study became a symbol of their mistreatment by the medical community, causing participants and their family members to be particularly distrustful of healthcare providers. This information is critical to this patient's care.

• Preceptor Pearls •

Consider the following culturally sensitive patient assessment questions:

- What do you think caused your illness or problem?

- What do you call your sickness or illness? How severe is it?

- What problems has your illness caused you?

- What kind of treatment do you think you should receive?

Adapted from Kleinman A. *Patients and Healers in the Context of Culture.* The American Medical Student Association. Berkeley, CA: University of California Press; 1980. Available at: http://www.amsa.org/programs/gpit/cultural.cfm. Accessed October 1, 2004.

Religion

If as preceptors we teach our students the importance of insightfully asking patients about their religious beliefs that may impact their care, we help make sure our students learn to provide appropriate recommendations that are suitable for their patients' beliefs. This will foster a trusting and respectful environment between the practitioner and the patient.

Students will invariably come across patients of various religious backgrounds regardless of their practice settings. The religious beliefs of patients are an important component to consider in a social assessment since they can impact the patient's healthcare. It is essential for the preceptor to teach students how to assess their patients for such beliefs, which helps ensure adequate care delivery while still being sensitive to patients' religious practices.

The content of some legend (prescription) and over-the counter medications are prohibited by followers of some religions This is an important aspect for the practitioner to be aware of and document appropriately in the patient record when considering recommending medication therapy, therapeutic changes, or dispensing medications, and in counseling patients. For instance, many Jehovah's Witness followers do not believe in taking any medications that contain human components. Thus, a discussion about individual beliefs of patients is important before prescribing or dispensing certain medications such as forms of epoetin and albumin.

Some followers of Hinduism, Buddhism, Islam, and Judaism have beliefs that incorporate dietary restrictions on meat products or on taking medications during fasting periods. A discussion on each patient's respective beliefs is important before prescribing many capsule formulations which include gelatin. In many instances it may be possible to use noncapsule dosage forms. Many capsules are now made with Kosher gelatin which many followers of Judaism and Islam would feel comfortable taking.

During Ramadan, adult Muslims are required to refrain from taking any food, beverages, or oral drugs between dawn and sunset. Because Ramadan can occur in any of the four seasons, the hours spent fasting can vary from 11–18 hours per day. The first meal is usually taken immediately after sunset and the second might be taken shortly before dawn. Many Muslim patients with chronic diseases insist on fasting even though they do not have to do so.[55] These patients may choose to change the time and dosing of their medications without seeking advice from their physician or pharmacist. Students should be able to inform their Muslim patients about when they should take their medication with regard to their altered food intake (before, with food, or after). A thorough patient history, including religious beliefs will allow the student to recommend and design a medication regimen which will be medically effective but sensitive to the patient's beliefs.

The Role of Family and Faith in Healthcare

The foundation of many cultural communities such as the Mexican and Mexican American communities is the nuclear family. Mexican and Mexican American families place value on having family members live close by, providing one another with mutual aid. Students should expect several family members to accompany a loved one to an appointment in a physician's office or clinic. This is particularly true following a hospital admission when family members eagerly await the outcome of the medical team's assessment or a surgical procedure.

No matter the social status or economic standing, caring for the elderly is considered the sole responsibility of the family in many cultures. Since pre-Hispanic times, family links in Mexico have been extremely strong, and as a result, caregiving of the elderly, sick, and poor is a socially recognized responsibility of the family, including members of the extended family.

• Preceptor Pearls •

In Hispanic and African American families, family can play an important role in assuring adherence to prescribed medication therapy or disease management.

It is estimated that 80% to 90% of Mexican Americans belong to the Roman Catholic church.[56] Many direct their prayers and religious promises to the Virgin of Guadalupe, the most popular religious symbol to Mexican Catholics. Patients may wish to have a religious symbol such as a rosary or other special amulet on them or near them during medical treatment. Students may encounter a patient bringing personal articles to various departments throughout a clinic or hospital that have a special meaning, such as ensuring the success of an examination or procedure.

Personal Space

Personal space is both an individual and cultural matter. As a general rule, patients tend to be very conservative about their personal space and modest about exposing their bodies to others— including health professionals. For example, Latin Americans may be hesitant to have pelvic examinations or even complete physicals. Students conducting a physical assessment should be aware of modesty concerns for both female and male patients.

Patients not familiar with the American healthcare system should be reassured and provided with appropriate information in a language they understand about what is happening and what is going to happen regarding their medical care. For many patients, support is most appropriately provided by family members. Preceptors should encourage students to consider incorporating family members whenever possible and allowing them to be present whenever possible.

Rather than objecting to something, Mexican Americans tend to use silence. A patient may appear to agree because of the cultural value of courtesy and respect.[57] Therefore, it is critical that students validate that a patient understands what is being communicated and provide an opportunity for open dialogue. Communicating respect is very important for the Mexican American when meeting someone, especially a healthcare professional. They in turn expect to be treated with respect until rapport is established over time and a less formal approach is acceptable.[58] Students should be cognizant of the tone of voice used, as well as eye contact, when communicating respect.

Providing Culturally Competent Care for Persons with Disabilities

Most of us will experience disability sometime in our lives, whether it be our own or that of a family member. Understanding the culture of disability makes it easier for the pharmacist and student to recognize barriers, make changes in your physical work environment, and prevent secondary conditions in your patients with disabilities. The definition of disability set forth in the Americans with Disabilities Act of 1990 (ADA) does not distinguish between type, severity, or duration of the disability. It states, "The term 'disability' means, with respect to an individual, (a) a physical or mental impairment that substantially limits one or more of the major life activities of such individual; (b) a record of such impairment; or (c) being regarded as having such an impairment."[59]

The ADA definition is an inclusive definition that tends to capture both the largest and broadest estimate of people with disabilities. It describes a disability as a condition that limits a person's ability to function in major life activities—including communication, walking, and self-care (such as feeding and dressing oneself)—and that is likely to continue indefinitely, resulting in the need for supportive services.

The United States Census Bureau also uses a broad definition of disability. Starting with the ADA definitions, the Census Bureau then expands its definition to identify people 16 years old and over as having disability if they meet any of the following criteria:

- used a wheelchair or were a long-term user of a cane, crutches, or a walker;
- had difficulty performing one or more functional activities, including seeing, hearing, speaking, lifting/carrying, using stairs, or walking;
- had difficulty with one or more activities of daily living (ADLs), including getting around inside the home, getting in or out of bed or a chair, bathing, dressing, eating, and toileting;
- had difficulty with one or more instrumental activities of daily living (IADLs), including going outside the home, keeping track of money and bills, preparing meals, doing light housework, taking prescription medication in the right amount at the right time, and using the telephone;
- had one or more specified conditions, including a learning disability, mental retardation or another developmental disability, Alzheimer's disease, or some other type of mental or emotional condition;
- were limited in their ability to do housework;
- were 16 to 67 years old and limited in their ability to work at a job or business; and were receiving federal benefits based on an inability to do work.

According to the 2000 Census there are an estimated 49.7 million persons in the U.S., or nearly 20% of the population, who are living with disabilities.[60] Persons with disabilities are individuals who have shared experiences and healthcare needs. Pharmacists and students should be familiar with their patients' limitations whether they be physical, sensory (vision or hearing), cognitive (following brain injury), or mental, in order to provide optimal care.

According to the American Association on Health and Disabilities (AAHD), for the millions of people with disabilities in the U.S., health maintenance and promotion often gets lost in the healthcare system quagmire. According to AAHD, people with disabilities are

- less likely to receive wellness screening,
- less likely to have access to specialists and follow-up care,
- more likely to be obese and a heavy smoker, and
- less likely to participate in an exercise program.[61]

• Preceptor Pearls •

When interacting with a person with a disability,

- identify yourself as a pharmacist/student and explain your role or purpose for the interaction.

- let the individual ask for assistance; don't assume the need; don't generalize or make assumptions without appropriate information.

- plan extra time for appointments when a patient uses an augmentative communication device.

- identify physically accessible rooms or facilities, with space to maneuver a wheelchair or scooter, or containing an adjustable examination table or chair.

- always address the individual (patient), not any other person or persons accompanying the patient, unless required because of cognition issues or problems.

- if the patient is cognitively impaired, it is important that you validate the patient's understanding by having him or her re-state the information you have provided. Also minimize noise or other distractions in the area or surrounding environment to allow for better comprehension by the patient.

- maintain and access community resources; develop educational information that can be used by persons with learning disabilities or sensory (visual, hearing, speech) impairments. Provide important educational materials (e.g., disease management) in written form; consider using a larger font, Braille, or an electronic format so that it can be accessed by a visually impaired person using a screen reader.

- learn how to use a text telephone or teletypewriter.

- provide disability-specific in-service education; keep abreast of the continuing advances in assistive technology and supportive equipment for people with disabilities.

In summary, preceptors need to educate students how to thoughtfully assess their patients' health beliefs, health-seeking behaviors, and general health knowledge. Coach them in the skill of gathering important patient information without being judgmental. Be quick to apologize, and accept responsibility for cultural missteps (e.g., calling a woman by her husband's last name—it is common for a woman to change her last name after marriage in the U.S.; this is not common practice outside the U.S.) Encourage students to read and learn more about the history and culture of the patients they are serving.

Preceptors can teach students the skills needed to be able to implement services that are accessible to and appropriate for diverse patient populations. Understanding the social and cultural background of the patients you serve and the environment that they live in is critical to providing quality patient care services. It is important to demonstrate to students how culturally competent clinical encounters result in more favorable outcomes, increase the satisfaction of the patient, and enhance the patient-provider experience. Being culturally competent will not only make you a more effective provider, but it will also make you a provider of choice.

References

1. Betancourt, JR. Cultural competence—marginal or mainstream movement? *N Engl J Med.* 2004:351(10)953–4.

2. Thomas, RR. *Building a House for Diversity.* New York, NY: AMACOM Publishers; 1999.

3. US Census Bureau. 2006 American community survey. Available at: http://factfinder.census.gov/serviet/ACCSSAFFFacts?_submenuld=factsheet_1&_sse=on. Accessed April 30, 2008.

4. AACP Institutional Research Report Series. *Profile of Pharmacy Students.* Alexandria, VA: American Association of Colleges of Pharmacy; Fall 2006.

5. Institute of Medicine (IOM). *The Nation's Compelling Interest: Ensuring Diversity in the Healthcare Workforce.* Washington, DC: National Academy Press; 2004.

6. US National Institutes of Health, National Cancer Institute. Health disparities defined. Available at: http://crchd.cancer.gov/definitions/defined.html. Accessed March 3, 2009.

7. United States of America. The minority health and health disparities research and education act of 2000. Public Law 106-525. *United States Code Congressional & Administrative News.* Eagan, MN: West Publishing; 2000:2498.

8. Office of Minority Health & Health Disparities (OMHD). Definitions of racial & ethnic populations. Available at: http://www.cdc.gov/omhd/Populations/definitionsREMP.htm. Accessed August 25, 2008.

9. American Cancer Society. Breast cancer death rates among black women not decreasing across all states. Available at: http://www.cancer.org/docroot/MED?content/MED_2_1x_Breast_Cancer_Death_Rates_Not_Decreasing_Across_All_States.asp. Accessed August 25, 2008.

10. Smedley BD, Stith AY, Nelson AR, eds. *Unequal Treatment: Confronting Racial and Ethnic Disparities in Healthcare.* Washington DC: National Academy Press; 2003.

11. The Sullivan Commission. Missing persons: minorities in the health professions—a report of the Sullivan Commission on diversity in the healthcare workforce, September 2004. Available at: http://www.sullivancommission.org. Accessed October 8, 2004.

12. *Fact Sheet: Racial and Ethnic Disparities.* Atlanta, GA; Centers for Disease Control and Prevention (CDC): April 2004.

13. Office of Minority Health and Health Disparities (OMHD). Eliminate disparities in diabetes. Available at: http://www.cdc.gov/omhd/AMH/factsheets/diabetes.htm. Accessed August 25, 2008.

14. Indian Health Service. *Facts on Indian Health Disparities.* Rockville, MD: Indian Health Service; September 2002.

15. Unites States Commission on Civil Rights. *The Healthcare Challenge: Acknowledging Disparity, Confronting Discrimination, and Ensuring Equality.* Washington, DC: Unites States Commission on Civil Rights; September 1999.

16. US Census Bureau. *Census 2000 Brief: Overview of Race and Hispanic Origin.* Washington, DC: US Census Bureau; 2000.

17. Kaiser Permanente. *A Provider's Handbook on Culturally Competent Care: Latino Population.* Oakland, CA: Kaiser Permanente National Diversity Council; 2001.

18. Doty MM, Holmgren AL. *Unequal Access: Insurance Instability Among Low-Income Workers and Minorities.* New York, NY: The Commonwealth Fund; April 2004.

19. Holahan J, Ghosh A. The Kaiser Commission on Medicaid and the Uninsured. *The Economic Downturn and Changes in Health Insurance Coverage,* 2000–2003. Washington, DC: The Henry J. Kaiser Family Foundation; September 2004.

20. The Kaiser Commission on Medicaid and the Uninsured. *The Uninsured and Their Access to Healthcare.* Washington, DC: The Henry J. Kaiser Family Foundation; October 2007.

21. *The Kaiser Commission on Medicaid and the Uninsured.* Washington, DC; August 2006.

22. Rosenbaum S, Sonosky C. *Policy Brief: Options for Assisting Uninsured Parents in Securing Basic Health Services.* New York, NY: The Commonwealth Fund; February 2002.

23. Reinburg S. Government picks up health tab of uninsured workers. *Washington Post.* May 2, 2008. Available at: http://www.washingtonpost.com/wp-dyn/content/article/2008/05/02/AR2008050201945.html.

24. The Kaiser Family Foundation and Health Research and Educational Trust. Employer health benefits: 2007 summary of findings. Available at: http://www.kff.org/insurance/7672/upload/Summary-of-Findings-EHBS-2007.pdf.

25. Regooulos LE, Trude S. Employers shift rising health care costs to workers: no long-term solution in sight. *Issue Brief Cent Stud Health Syst Change.* 2004 May;(83):1–4.

26. The Kaiser Commission on Medicaid and the Uninsured. *Health Insurance Coverage and Access to Care Among Latinos.* Washington, DC: The Henry J. Kaiser Family Foundation; June 2000.

27. The Kaiser Commission on Medicaid and the Uninsured. *Medicaid and the Uninsured.* Washington, DC: The Henry J. Kaiser Family Foundation; March 2008.

28. Grantmakers in Health, Washington DC. Strategies for reducing racial and ethnic disparities in health. *Issue Brief (Grantmakers Health).* 2000; May 18(5):1–36.

29. The Kaiser Commission on Medicaid and the Uninsured. *Health Insurance Coverage and Access to Care Among American Indians and Alaska Natives.* Washington, DC: The Henry J. Kaiser Family Foundation; June 2000.

30. The Kaiser Commission on Medicaid and the Uninsured. *American Indians and Alaska Natives: Health Coverage and Access to Care.* Washington, DC: The Henry J. Kaiser Family Foundation; February 2004.

31. The Kaiser Commission on Medicaid and the Uninsured. *Health Insurance Coverage and Access to Care Among African Americans.* Washington, DC: The Henry J. Kaiser Family Foundation; June 2000.

32. The Henry J. Kaiser Family Foundation. *Women's Health Policy Facts: Women's Health Insurance Coverage.* Washington, DC: The Henry J. Kaiser Family Foundation; December 2007.

33. The Henry J. Kaiser Family Foundation. *Racial and Ethnic Disparities in Women's Health Coverage and Access to Care: Findings from the 2001 Kaiser Women's Health Survey.* Washington, DC: The Henry J. Kaiser Family Foundation; March 2004.

34. The Kaiser Commission on Medicaid and the Uninsured. *Health Insurance Coverage and Access to Care Among Asian Americans and Pacific Islanders.* Washington, DC: The Henry J. Kaiser Family Foundation; June 2000.

35. The Henry J. Kaiser Family Foundation. *Trends in Health Care Costs and Spending.* Washington, DC: The Henry J. Kaiser Family Foundation; September 2007.

36. Banthin JS, Bernard DM. Changes in financial burdens for health care: national estimates for the population younger than 65 years, 1996 to 2003. *JAMA.* 2006;296(22):2712–9.

37. Mary JH, Cunningham PJ. Tough trade-offs: medical bills, family finances and access to care. *Issue Brief Cent Stud Health Syst Change.* 2004 Jun;(85):1–4.

38. Tu HT. Rising health costs, medical debt and chronic conditions. *Issue Brief Cent Stud Health Syst Change.* 2004 Sep;(88):1–5.

39. US Department of Health and Human Services, Office of Disease Prevention and Health Promotion. *Healthy People 2010: Understanding and Improving Health.* Rockville, MD: US Department of Health and Human Services; November 2000.

40. Kalichman, SC, Benotsch E, Suarez T, et al. Health literacy and health-related knowledge among persons living with HIV/AIDS. *Am J Prev Med.* 2000;18(4):325–31.

41. US Department of Education, National Center for Education Statistics. National assessment of adult literacy (NAAL). Available at: http://nces.ed.gov/naal/kf_demographics.asp. Accessed August 26, 2008.

42. Kirsch IS, Jungeblut A, Jenkins L, et al. *Adult Literacy in America: A First Look at the Results of the National Adult Survey (NALS).* Washington, DC: US Department of Education, National Center for Education Statistics; 1993.

43. Parker R, Williams MV, Davis T. *Low Health Literacy—You Can't Tell by Looking* [videotape]. Chicago, IL: American Medical Association Foundation; 1999.

44. US Department of Education, National Center for Education Statistics. National assessment of adult literacy (NAAL): a first look at the literacy of America's adults in the 21st century. Available at: http://nces.ed.gov/NAAL/PDF/2006470.pdf. Accessed August 26, 2008.

45. Baker DW, Parker RM, Williams MV, et al. The healthcare experience of patients with low literacy. *Arch Fam Med.* 1996;5(6):329–34.

46. Williams MV, Baker DW, Parker RM, et al. Relationship of functional health literacy to patients' knowledge of their chronic disease: a study of patients with hypertension and diabetes. *Arch Intern Med.* 1998;158(2):166–72.

47. Youmans SL, Schillinger D. Functional health literacy and medication use: the pharmacist's role. *Ann Pharmacother.* 2003;37(11):1726–9.

48. National Center for Cultural Competence. Conceptual frameworks/models, guiding values and principles. Available at: http://gucchd.georgetown,edu//ncc/. Accessed June 18, 2004.

49. Cohen E, Goode TD. *Rationale for Cultural Competence in Primary Healthcare. Policy Brief 1.* Washington, DC: National Center for Cultural Competence; 1999.

50. Kaiser Permanente. *A Provider's Handbook on Culturally Competent Care: Asian and Pacific Islander Population.* 2nd ed. Oakland, CA; Kaiser Permanente National Diversity Council; 2001.

51. Kaiser Permanente. *A Provider's Handbook on Culturally Competent Care: Latino Population.* 2nd ed. Oakland, CA; Kaiser Permanente National Diversity Council; 2001.

52. US Department of Health and Human Services, Office of Minority Health. *National Standards on Culturally and Linguistically Appropriate Services (CLAS) in Healthcare Final Report.* Rockville, MD: Office of Minority Health; 2001.

53. Kaczmarczyk JM, Burke A. *Complementary and Alternative Medicine Issues in Serving Diverse Populations. Module 7 of Cultural Competence in the Clinical Care of Patients with Diabetes and Cardiovascular Disease.* Washington, DC: Health Resources and Services Administration, Bureau of Primary Healthcare, and Institute for Healthcare Improvement; 2003.

54. US Department of Health and Human Services (US DHHS). (2003a). *Complementary and Alternative Medicine: Issues in Serving Diverse Populations.* Draft curriculum module 5 for Cultural Competence in the Clinical Care Model Project. Washington, DC: Health Resources and Services Administration, Bureau of Primary Healthcare; 2001.

55. Aadil N, Houti IE, Moussamih S. Drug intake during Ramadan. *BMJ.* 2004;329:778–82.

56. de Paula T, Lagana K, Gonzalez-Ramirez L. Mexican Americans. In: Lipson JG, Dibble SL, Minarik PA, eds. *Culture and Nursing Care.* San Francisco, CA: UCSF Nursing Press; 1996.

57. Murillo N. The Mexican American family. In: Hernandez CA, Haug MJ, Wagner NN, eds. *Chicanos: Social and Psychological Perspectives*. St. Louis, MO: Mosby; 1978:15–25.

58. Kuipers J. Mexican Americans. In: Giger J, Davidhizar R, eds. *Transcultural Nursing: Assessment and Intervention*. St. Louis, MO: Mosby Year Book; 2004.

59. American with Disabilities Act. (P.L. 101-336, Sec.). Available at: http://www.ada.gov/pubs/ada.htm. Accessed March 2, 2009.

60. US Census Bureau. *Disability Status: 2000*. Washington DC:US Department of Commerce, Economics and Statistics Administration; 2000.

61. American Association on Health and Disability. A health care solution: disability-competent health systems. Available at. http://www.aahd.us/page.php?pname=publications/newsletters/2006/fall/bestPractices2&P. Accessed August 27, 2008.

Additional Resources

Betancourt, JR. *The Impact of Race/Ethnicity, Culture, and Class on Clinical Decision-Making. Module 4 of Cultural Competence in the Clinical Care of Patients with Diabetes and Cardiovascular Disease (2002)*. Washington, DC: Health Resources and Services Administration, Bureau of Primary Healthcare, and Institute for Healthcare Improvement; 2003.

Ferguson JA, Weinberger GR, Westmoreland LA, et al. Racial disparity in cardiac decision making. *Arch Internal Med*. 1998;158(13):1450–3.

Flaskerud JH, Uman G. Directions for AIDS education for Hispanic women based on analyses of survey findings. *Public Health Rep*. 1993;108(3):298–304.

Frederick Schneiders Research. *Perceptions of How Race and Ethnic Background Affect Medical Care: Highlights from Focus Groups*. Menlo Park, CA: The Henry J. Kaiser Family Foundation; 1999.

Gordon AK. Deterrents to access and service for Blacks and Hispanics: the Medicare hospice benefit, healthcare utilization, and cultural barriers. *Hospice J*. 1995;10(2):65–83.

McKenzie K. Racism and health. *Br Med J*. 2003;326:65–6.

Morales LS, Cunningham WE, Brown JA, et al. Are Latinos less satisfied with communication by healthcare providers? *J Gen Intern Med*. 1999;14(7):409–17.

National Center for Cultural Competence. Conceptual frameworks/models, guiding values and principles. Available at: http://www11.georgetown.edu/research/gucchd/nccc/foundations/frameworks.html. Accessed April 15, 2009.

Peterson ED, Wright SM, Daley J, et al. Racial variation in cardiac procedure use and survival following acute myocardial infarction in the department of veterans affairs. *JAMA*. 1994;271(15):1175–80.

Program for multicultural health. University of Michigan Health System Web site. Available at: http://www.med.umich.edu/Multicultural/ccp/culcomp.htm. Accessed April 15, 2009.

Tocher TM, Larson E. Quality of diabetes care for non-English speaking patients: a comparative study. *West J Med*. 1998;168:504–11.

Uba L. Cultural barriers to healthcare for Southeast Asian refugees. *Public Health Rep*. 1992;107(5):544–8.

US Department of Health and Human Services, Office of Minority Health. Think cultural health: bridging the health care gap through cultural competency continuing education programs. Available at: http://www.thinkculturalhealth.org. Accessed April 15, 2009.

van Ryn M, Burke J. The effect of patient race and socio-economic status on physicians' perceptions of patients. *Soc Sci Med.* 2000;50:813–28.

Wagner TH, Guendelman S. Healthcare utilization among Hispanics: findings from the 1994 minority health survey. *Am J Manag C.* 2000;6:355–64.

If I can dream, I can act. And if I can act, I can become.
Poh Yu Khing

Chapter 9

Professionalism and Professional Socialization

Edward Stemley, Kevin Purcell, John E. Murphy, David Lorms

Chapter Outline

Learning Objectives

- Describe the responsibility of a pharmacist to exude excellent moral and ethical character.

- Provide an overview of the interdisciplinary and multifaceted approach to professionalism.

- Explain the importance of setting clear expectations regarding professionalism.

- Identify valuable resources to reinforce preceptor teaching and modeling of professionalism.

- Describe the impact that leadership in professional organizations has on the pharmacy profession and the patients it serves.

- Define the intrinsic and extrinsic value that volunteerism has on pharmacy professionals and the community.

- Describe the value system and compassion needed by pharmacists to continually improve pharmacy practice and ultimately patient care.

Preceptors play a crucial role in the transition of pharmacy students to pharmacy professionals. This opportunity for experiential training and mentoring serves as the mortar needed to strengthen the strong foundation of pharmacy knowledge and skills set forth by didactic learning. This chapter will reach beyond the realms of the function of the pharmacist in an attempt to define the behavior in which these responsibilities should be practiced.

Professionalism

"The practice of pharmacy is not about dispensing drugs, but about taking care of patients."[1]

Being a pharmacist goes far beyond merely graduating from pharmacy school, passing the NAPLEX and MPJE, and having an active pharmacy license. By the same token, being a professional goes far beyond merely becoming a member of a profession. Certainly, pharmacists do dispense drugs, but our purpose as healthcare professionals is to take care of patients. Pharmacists help patients, physicians, and other healthcare providers with the management of the patient's drug therapy and overall health. A pharmacist must understand what it means to be a healthcare professional before he or she can successfully serve that purpose. The concept of being a pharmacist ultimately refers to embodying all of the hallmark qualities and characteristics (e.g., commitment, self-sacrifice, pride, knowledge, skills, abilities, values, attitudes, beliefs, and behaviors) of a pharmacy professional.

To understand the role of professionalism in pharmacy practice, it is important first to understand the concepts of *profession*, *professional*, *professionalism*, and *professionalization*. A *profession* is an occupation whose members share 10 common characteristics (Box 9.1), and a *professional* is a member of a profession who displays 10 common traits (Box 9.2); therefore, *professionalism* is the active demonstration of the traits of a professional.[2] Finally, *professionalization* (professional socialization) is the process of instilling students with a profession's attitudes, values, and behaviors so that they learn to become professionals.[2]

Box 9.1 • Definition of a Profession

Profession: An occupation whose members share 10 common characteristics.

1. Prolonged specialized training in a body of abstract knowledge
2. A service orientation
3. An ideology based on the original faith professed by members
4. An ethic that is binding on the practitioners
5. A body of knowledge unique to the members
6. A set of skills that forms the technique of the profession
7. A guild of those entitled to practice the profession
8. Authority granted by society in the form of licensure and certification
9. A recognized setting where the profession is practiced
10. A theory of societal benefits derived from the ideology

Developed by the American Pharmaceutical Association Academy of Students of Pharmacy and the American Association of Colleges of Pharmacy Council of Deans Task Force on Professionalism.

Box 9.2 • Definition of a Professional

Professional: A member of a profession who displays the following 10 traits.

1. Knowledge and skills of a profession
2. Commitment to self-improvement of skills and knowledge
3. Service orientation
4. Pride in the profession
5. Covenantal relationship with the client
6. Creativity and innovation
7. Conscience and trustworthiness
8. Accountability for his/her work
9. Ethically sound decision making
10. Leadership

Developed by the American Pharmaceutical Association Academy of Students of Pharmacy and the American Association of Colleges of Pharmacy Council of Deans Task Force on Professionalism.

Professionalization of students requires a spectrum of activities over a long period of time in a diverse set of environments (e.g., classroom, practice sites, professional society settings, and community service organization settings) that positively influence their professional perspectives and development. Many people are coresponsible for the professionalization process, including students, faculty and administrative staff, pharmacy practitioners, pharmacy technicians, and other healthcare professionals.[3] Preceptors need to recognize and appreciate the important role that they play in the professionalization process through role modeling and establishing mentoring relationships.[2,3]

Preceptors may facilitate a discussion on the topic of professionalism with students in a variety of ways and stimulate them to engage in a process of self-assessment, self-reflection, and self-transformation. Preceptors can point out both positive and negative examples of professionalism in patient care, pharmacy operations, and professional and business relationships. Case studies and role-playing exercises may supplement real-life situations that occur during the pharmacy practice experience. Preceptors can share their thoughts and feelings on professionalism and some of their personal experiences from their own professionalization process. Preceptors can also discuss with students what they do to continue to grow and develop as pharmacy practitioners and health professionals and to attain a level of excellence as patient care providers, teachers, researchers, managers, and/or leaders. Lastly, preceptors can express their professional pride they have about being pharmacists and what it has meant to them—the relationships they have formed with patients and colleagues, the care they have provided, and the difference they have made in people's lives. There is nothing like a true hero story to reinforce the desired pharmacy culture, set a high bar of achievement, and inspire others to outdo what has been done and raise the bar even higher.

There are several important documents that preceptors can use to facilitate a discussion of professionalism and to reinforce professional ideals. Pharmacy students recite the Pledge of Professionalism (Box 9.3) at a white coat ceremony during their first professional year and the Oath of a Pharmacist (Box 9.4) at their graduation ceremony. The Code of Ethics for Pharmacists (see Chapter 7) states the principles that form the fundamental basis of the roles and responsibilities of pharmacists. Pharmacy students should be familiar with and adhere to all of these critical works that define what it means to be a pharmacist and a healthcare professional. All provide guidance to those on a lifelong journey to become the best pharmacists they can be. These documents may not encompass everything that one should know about pharmacy professionalism, but they do include reference to all of the key elements of professionalism, including honor/integrity, altruism/advocacy, duty/service, responsibility/accountability, respect for others, compassion/empathy, communication/collaboration, self-awareness/knowledge of limits, and a commitment to lifelong learning and professional growth and development.[4,5] Additionally, preceptors can discuss with students the importance of a positive attitude, professional attire and appearance, punctuality, organization, time management, follow-through, and openness to constructive criticism.

Box 9.3 • Pledge of Professionalism

As a student of pharmacy, I believe there is a need to build and reinforce a professional identity founded on integrity, ethical behavior, and honor. This development, a vital process in my education, will help ensure that I am true to the professional relationship I establish between myself and society as I become a member of the pharmacy community. Integrity must be an essential part of my everyday life, and I must practice pharmacy with honesty and commitment to service.

To accomplish this goal of professional development, I, as a student of pharmacy, should adhere to the following:

DEVELOP a sense of loyalty and duty to the profession of pharmacy by being a builder of community, one able and willing to contribute to the well-being of others and one who enthusiastically accepts the responsibility and accountability for membership in the profession.

FOSTER professional competency through lifelong learning. I must strive for high ideals, teamwork, and unity within the profession in order to provide optimal patient care.

SUPPORT my colleagues by actively encouraging personal commitment to the Oath of Maimonides and a Code of Ethics as set forth by the profession.

INCORPORATE into my life and practice, dedication to excellence. This will require an ongoing reassessment of personal and professional values.

MAINTAIN the highest ideals and professional attributes to ensure and facilitate the covenantal relationship required of the pharmaceutical caregiver.

The profession of pharmacy is one that demands adherence to a set of rigid, ethical standards. These high ideals are necessary to ensure the quality of care extended to the patients I serve. As a student of pharmacy, I believe this does not start with graduation; rather, it begins with my membership in this professional college community. Therefore, I must strive to uphold these standards as I advance toward full membership in the profession of pharmacy.

Developed and adopted by the American Pharmaceutical Association Academy of Students of Pharmacy and the American Association of Colleges of Pharmacy Council of Deans Task Force on Professionalism, June 26, 1994.

Box 9.4 • Oath of a Pharmacist

At this time, I vow to devote my professional life to the service of all humankind through the profession of pharmacy.

I will consider the welfare of humanity and relief of human suffering my primary concerns.

I will apply my knowledge, experience, and skills to the best of my ability to assure optimal drug therapy outcomes for the patients I serve.

Box 9.4 • Oath of a Pharmacist (cont'd)

I will keep abreast of developments and maintain professional competency in my profession of pharmacy.

I will maintain the highest principles of moral, ethical, and legal conduct.

I will embrace and advocate change in the profession of pharmacy that improves patient care.

I take these vows voluntarily with the full realization of the responsibility with which I am entrusted by the public.

Developed by the American Pharmaceutical Association Academy of Students of Pharmacy/American Association of Colleges of Pharmacy Council of Deans (APhA-ASP/AACP-COD) Task Force on Professionalism; June 26, 1994.

Preceptors need to set clear expectations regarding professionalism at the beginning of the pharmacy practice experience. A discussion of professional expectations and examples of intolerable behaviors can be included in the orientation session. Preceptors should also provide periodic formative feedback on the professionalism of students throughout the pharmacy practice experience. Optimally, preceptors will have the ability to formally assess the professionalism of students as part of the final evaluation at the end of the pharmacy practice experience. Students should also have the opportunity to assess their own professionalism as part of the evaluation process. Then, if there is a discrepancy between the preceptors' rating and the students' self-evaluation, preceptors can have a final discussion on professionalism with students that examines the difference in their perspectives and stimulates deeper reflection on the part of the students.

• Preceptor Pearls •

Set clear expectations regarding professionalism at the beginning of the pharmacy practice experience.

Getting to know and working with others are good ways for students to enhance their professionalization and their understanding of the role of pharmacists in the healthcare system and the community. Communication with patients is absolutely necessary for most pharmacy practice experiences. Students need to learn how to develop pharmacist-patient relationships based on mutual trust, respect, and commitment. Also, spending time with other healthcare professionals, either one-on-one or as part of a patient care team, can be very beneficial. Preceptors can take students along and get them involved in any community service or professional society activities in which the preceptors participate. Community service activities can provide students with a broader understanding of issues faced and enhance their cultural competency. Professional society activities can increase student identification with the pharmacy profession and provide students with a network of peers.

Teaching pharmacy students about important principles of the pharmacy profession and showing students how to live them is a critical responsibility of preceptors. Remember that the messenger is often as important as the message, and the two must in harmony or students will become confused or cynical. Preceptors need to lead by example and create an atmosphere that promotes professionalism, fosters lifelong learning, and nurtures professional growth and development. This can be challenging at times in some practice settings due to work-related and marketplace factors, as well as to general societal influences. It is imperative that preceptors communicate these challenges and related approaches for resolution with students as a part of the learning process. Pharmacists entering the workplace will require the knowledge and skills necessary to assess their professional environment for work-related and marketplace challenges and the leadership ability necessary to develop related plans for resolution. It requires a team effort to maintain a professional image and practice environment in any pharmacy setting. Pharmacists, technicians, and students are all part of that team and contribute to establishing and maintaining a climate of professionalism.

The Role of Participation in Pharmacy Professional Organizations

The Importance of Preceptor Involvement

It is hard to argue that a profession can get along well without leaders, though "leaving it up to someone else" is the most often noted outcome when it comes time to volunteer for leadership opportunities. The 80:20 rule (80% of the work will be done by 20% of the people) certainly seems to apply in many professional organizations, pharmacy included. However, preceptors may not rest among the silent majority when it comes to participation in professional pharmacy organizations. They have accepted positions as role models who "must be committed to developing professionalism and fostering leadership in students and to serving as mentors and positive role models for students" as well as being "committed to their organization, professional societies, and the community."[6] By the nature of the job, preceptors are already among the 20% making things happen for the future of the profession when it comes to education.

The ASHP Statement on Professionalism says that "Professional education and advancing standards of practice can only be achieved through a profession's *collective efforts* (emphasis added); pharmacists therefore commit themselves to serve not only their patients but also their profession."[7] The statement further emphasizes characteristics of a professional that include service orientation, pride in and service to the profession, and leadership, among others.

Since students will mimic the behaviors of those people whom they identify as successful, it is up to you to provide the model of a successful practitioner and leader of the profession, no matter what your role in the profession might be.

It is, therefore, quite fortunate that participating in professional organizations can add so much to your career as a pharmacist and preceptor role model. For example, as your career progresses, you may realize that every volunteer effort was at least as beneficial to you personally or professionally as to the organization. One author has even commented that these opportunities are nearly akin to thievery.[8] In her excellent "Success Skills" series on leadership and development, ASHP past-president Sara White frequently stresses the value of participating in organizations, in serving as a mentor, and in finding a mentor for yourself.[9-11]

• Preceptor Pearls •

Take the time to participate in professional organizations and also to share the reasons why participation is so important for the future of the profession. Doing so can provide a strong influence to students under your care and guidance.

The notion of gaining from activities outside of traditional studying, such as active participation in organizations, is well-known in academia.[12-14] It has been estimated that much of the cognitive development of college students comes from their activities outside the classroom (cocurricular and extracurricular activities).[15] An example of this is the opportunity to discuss issues and academics during dormitory life that leads to enhanced cognitive understanding, much like the opportunities that occur from meeting with colleagues at a professional meeting. Further, participation in student organizations has been specifically identified as playing an integral role in the educational process.[14]

An important component of your development as a professionally competent clinician, manager, educator, business person, and preceptor also comes, to a significant degree, from activities outside of the daily practice as a pharmacist. Participation in the activities of a professional organization can be one of the great ways to help continue the development of many important job and life skills. The profession needs people who are dedicated to advancing its causes, and becoming a preceptor is an important commitment in the creation of future generations of colleagues.

Participation for the preceptor can be described as a hierarchy, with many of the elements occurring at the same time. Below are activities you should consider in the development of your role as preceptor so you can be the best role model for your students.

- Join the organization and pay dues. (This is critically important as member numbers allow the organization to have a voice.)
- Attend meetings and make your voice heard.
- Volunteer for committees/task forces/special projects.[9]
- Chair committees.
- Participate in legislative activities.
- Give presentations and present posters.
- Run for office.

Active participation can generate benefits for you that may then be demonstrated to the students. This allows the profession to benefit now and in the future.

The Importance of Student Involvement

As might be expected, many of the reasons students should begin getting involved in professional organizations during their college years (and certainly after graduation) are the same as those for preceptors. For one, involved students are more likely to see the value of the profession to them and the importance of promoting the profession for their own future. Other important reasons include the following:

- Enhancing professionalism
- Creating a professional network
- Developing future leaders
- Developing an attitude of interest in the profession
- Promoting community service
- Instilling a feeling of obligation to the profession
- Establishing a common spirit among members of the organizations

Many students will come to their experiential education settings with a wealth of experience in student organizations and college governance.[15] However, it is quite common for those students who were active in student organizations to become less active in their pharmacy practice experience year and even less so once they become practicing professionals. The professional organizations therefore work very hard to attract graduates to their fold with programs such as Young Practitioners and with reduced dues for the first year or more after graduation. Unfortunately, these incentives are only partially effective, thus creating the need for preceptors to reinforce the value of participation in professional organizations.

Selected Modeling Suggestions

- Discuss the value of participating in professional organizations with students.
- Invite your students to a local professional meeting, or even better, take them with you.
- If feasible, make it a rotation requirement that students attend at least one meeting in a professional organization and report back to you on what occurred during the meeting.
- Introduce students to influential pharmacists and potential employers at meetings.
- Have the students recognized as new attendees during meetings.
- Bring the students to a committee meeting.
- Help the students get on a committee as a student member, when it is possible.
- Sponsor students. Pay part of the students' attendance fee at a pharmacy meeting or part of their dues to a professional organization. Even a small subsidy demonstrates clear commitment on your part. Tell them why you are providing the sponsorship. Encourage other pharmacists to sponsor students as well.

Didactic Opportunities

- Conduct a study session on a professional organization. Have the students compare and contrast selected national organizations (mission, vision, services).
- Discuss the reasons why people join organizations beginning with the general reasons (e.g., continuing education, networking, legislative representation) and then personalize to your reasons.
- Assign readings and discuss the history of various organizations such as the American Society of Health-System Pharmacists and the American Pharmacists Association (articles are printed in most issues of the *Journal of the American Pharmacists Association*).[16]

- Assign and discuss readings on leadership and professionalism such as the "Success Skill" series by Sara White and the ASHP Statement on Professionalism.

- Give the students a sense of the profession's leaders (e.g., read and discuss the Harvey A.K. Whitney Award Lectures or articles about individual leaders).[17,18]

- Explore international pharmacy organizations such as The International Pharmaceutical Federation (FIP; see http://www.fip.org/) and the International Pharmaceutical Students' Federation (IPSF; see http://www.ipsf.org/). Discuss how pharmacy in other countries may affect practice in the United States and what our role is in helping promote pharmacy in other countries.

These are but a few of the many reasons why it is important for preceptors and students to be involved in professional organizations and why you can make a difference in the lives of students when it comes to advancing the profession. You have already made an extremely important contribution to the future of our profession by serving as a preceptor. Participating in professional organizations allows you to continue to grow personally and professionally and allows many opportunities to inspire students and to provide mentoring on what is needed in our future generations of pharmacists. Your modeling of the importance of professionalism will go a long way toward creating future leaders in the profession and you will likely find the experiences to be well worth your while; it is very satisfying to see students achieve goals and move forward in the profession. Perhaps you too will create the kind of memories that were described in a recent "Reflections" article by a pharmacy student who likened her experience with a mentor to standing in the shadow of a "pharmacy giant."[19] We all can leave a big shadow through our efforts to advance the profession and to provide mentoring to our students.

• Preceptor Pearls •

Participating in professional organizations allows you to continue to grow personally and professionally and allows many opportunities to inspire students.

Community Service: The Broader Role of Professionalism

Other parts of this text have addressed the various roles of the preceptor in direct relationship to the students whom they precept and to the practice of pharmacy. By addressing professionalism and professional socialization, this chapter recognizes an underappreciated but essential overarching aspect of the pharmacist in society and in their communities.

As much as pharmacists play an important role in public health policy and its implementation and development, it is imperative that students see themselves actively engaged in this important activity from the beginning of their careers. Regardless of practice setting, pharmacy as a profession—through the involvement of its individual practitioners—has been instrumental in its support for a variety of public health issues at the local state and national levels. In order to fulfill obligations to their communities, preceptors have a responsibility to ensure students have broad exposure and see themselves as integral to the success of volunteer service in any at any level.

Preceptors have opportunities to challenge students to find their own voice in community with others by virtue of their own community involvement. For this exposure to result in a longer term commitment to service it will be important that the preceptor ensure a broad overview, that prompts the student to be responsible for their own choice. Pharmacists across the country participate as volunteers in a variety of general activities within their community as well as health-focused organizations. They serve as elected leaders in their cities and at the state level, and volunteer in clinics in their inner cities. Their participation and personal leadership development in these activities serves to move the broader community agenda forward. The success of their experience encourage others to be more engaged in everyday activities. Essential to a successful exposure to community service is an introduction to the legislative process and its leaders through a lobby day experience.

An example of the valuable role an active pharmacist can play came from was Dennis Penña. His service on the state board of the American Heart Association aided the development of community education programs. As a state legislator he provided essential links to the legislative and regulatory decision-makers formerly inaccessible to this organization's community leaders.

To be certain, students will not have the depth of interest or capacity needed as they come directly from school; however, the preceptor's leadership role leads them to find their own niche in the world of volunteerism—a niche that they will be able to grow with as they progress in the profession.

Tom Peters, in his treatise *The BrandYou 50*, suggests that one can assume responsibilities for many of those smaller, less glamorous tasks in organizations and turn them into success steps for a career.[20] These tasks can be found in churches, almost any nationally focused health agency, or the public school system as Phil Johnson, a past president of the Florida Society of Health-System Pharmacists, found. Johnson uncovered a simple truth that the school systems are a large provider of healthcare to our children. He became the chief volunteer leader for a nationally known and respected program called Medication Use in Schools sponsored by FSHP.

Students often wonder, "What's in it for me?" You, as a preceptor, bring an understanding of the phrase, "Volunteer service is the rent we pay for taking up space in our communities." Your example shows how the pay for volunteer work translates into a sense of accomplishment and feeling of achievement and how the exposure to new audiences (or activities) can engage their pharmacy spirit and provide recognition. Then and only then, can the essential threads in the warp and weft of the community fabric in our professional and public lives be strengthened.

Students' appreciation for their time and effort can be engaged by illustrating how their skills in communications, facilitation, planning, speaking, writing, or delegating (when paired with character-istics of accessibility, team play, goal-orientation, vision, sense of success, and personal commitment to a cause) can indeed make a significant and positive impact on their community.

Pointing students to opportunities of interest can be easy. It is important for the preceptor to help them see a personal stake in their first few ventures to ensure the experience is a positive and profound one. Aside from the major health agencies, smaller community groups also need assistance. As a preceptor, you might consider focusing their interest as it warrants to the political process for both state and federal issues and elections. This last group of opportunities will undoubtedly open their eyes to further interest in societal environmental factors that impact their profession.

• Preceptor Pearls •

When helping your students find community service opportunities, don't forget the smaller community groups.

No matter the students' practice interests, there are one or two professional organizations that support their short- and long-term professional development. It is these groups, where their professional commitment is developed, that prepare them for a career rich in professional connections and community. A recent study by ASAE & The Center for Association Leadership identified four distinct patterns of engagement based on the types of activities in which volunteers from the sponsoring organizations were involved.[21] **Local Leaders** focus effort on local board and committee service, mentoring and membership recruitment. **Writers** are likely to be the subject matter experts and engage in writing and reviews of publications and professional papers. **Teachers**, while minimally engaged in other areas, are important sources of professional advice, mentoring and recruitment. **Shapers** are involved in many areas of their organizations. Preceptors may benefit from examining their own pattern as they develop a culture of voluntarism among their students.

Pharmacy Spirit

Pharmacy spirit is the energy, loyalty, dedication, and courage that push forward the frontiers of pharmacy practice. Pharmacy spirit is the heart and driving force behind providing and improving patient care. Pharmacy spirit is the enthusiasm, determination, and commitment, as well as the love, compassion, and kindness required for providing the best possible patient care. It is the soul of the pharmacy profession. Having pharmacy spirit symbolizes the ultimate commitment to the pharmacy oath, and therefore to the profession of pharmacy and to the public.[22,23]

Pharmacy spirit describes the humanistic qualities, character, and strong will that are necessary to form good patient-pharmacist relationships, to effectively practice the art and science of pharmacy, to continuously improve patient care, and to advance the pharmacy profession. It is the force of this spirit that all outstanding pharmacy practitioners and leaders feel and draw on. Having pharmacy spirit gives meaning to the practice of pharmacy by putting into broader context the little things that are done as part of routine daily work and that make a difference in the lives of others. Instilling pharmacy spirit into students is the culmination of precepting and mentoring. Exemplary preceptors and mentors radiate pharmacy spirit and energize their preceptees and mentees to be the best pharmacists they can be and to make a positive impact on the lives of the people they serve. Having and radiating pharmacy spirit and instilling pharmacy spirit into others may be the quintessential expression of pharmacy professionalism. Ultimately, when students fully appreciate and use the power of pharmacy spirit, the torch of leadership is passed from one generation to the next. Leadership is central to the concept of pharmacy spirit. Power as it relates to pharmacy spirit is no different from power as it relates to positive thinking. In both cases, your inspiration and success come from a specific way of thinking and viewing the world.

• Preceptor Pearls •

Use your own pharmacy spirit to instill pharmacy spirit into others and to fully express your own professionalism.

As role models for students, preceptors must lead by example and display pharmacy spirit and embody its elements (Box 9.5). Preceptors can show care and respect for others by having compassion and sensitivity and helping them maintain their dignity and self-esteem. Preceptors can demonstrate pharmacy spirit by putting the needs of patients first and by understanding the impact of their own and others' actions on their patients. Preceptors can demonstrate how to take action and assume responsibility for the care of patients by being alert, having a high index of suspicion, and resolving any actual or potential drug-related problems and any other healthcare-related issues that are identified and could adversely affect patient outcomes. Preceptors can display a drive to achieve excellence as practitioners by trying out new ways of doing things in order to advance the practice of pharmacy and improve patient care. Preceptors can discuss with students the need to renew and reinvent themselves through a continual process of self-assessment, self-reflection, and self-transformation. Preceptors can talk with students about the history of their profession, important pharmacy traditions, and distinguished pharmacists who led the way in the past. Above all, preceptors must have a passion for what they do, a positive attitude, and a true desire to serve the public and to help students grow and develop.

Box 9.5 • The Elements of Pharmacy Spirit

P rofessionalism

H eart

A ction

R enewal

M entoring

A dventure

C aring

Y earning

S ervice

P assion

I deals

R esponsibility

I magination

T radition

Ultimately, preceptors want their students to posses and exhibit pharmacy spirit. Preceptors can encourage their students and acknowledge and praise them when they demonstrate their ability to help advance the practice of pharmacy and improve patient care. People have a tendency to rise to the level of expectation and belief that others have in them (the Pygmalion effect). Communication between student and preceptor is a key ingredient in the learning process as it addresses the potential relationship barrier that can be the result of generational gaps. Preceptors can talk with students about each other's experiences with patient care, pharmacy practice, and leadership and stimulate reflective thinking and learning about what it means to be a pharmacist, a healthcare professional, and a leader. Finally, preceptors can recognize and reward their students when they show pharmacy spirit. For example, preceptors could present a pharmacy spirit certificate to students who radiate and exemplify pharmacy spirit (Figure 9.1). This simple but significant gesture may have a long-lasting impact on students' professional growth and development. May the pharmacy spirit be with you!

Pharmacy spirit is the energy, loyalty, dedication, and courage that pushes forward the frontiers of pharmacy practice. Pharmacy spirit is the heart and driving force behind providing and improving patient care. Pharmacy spirit is the enthusiasm, determination, and commitment, as well as the love, compassion, and kindness required for providing the best possible patient care. Pharmacy spirit is the soul of the pharmacy profession. Having pharmacy spirit symbolizes the ultimate commitment to the Pharmacy Oath, and therefore to the profession of pharmacy and to the public.

This distinguished *PHARMACY SPIRIT AWARD*
is presented to

_____

on the __th day of _____ in the year ____.

Like a lighthouse ever shining light into the night to guide ships safely along their journey, you act as a beacon for the pharmacy profession by expressing pharmacy spirit and by leading pharmacists in the advancement of the practice of pharmacy and the care of patients.

_____

Preceptor's Name
Preceptor's Title
Preceptor's Practice Site

Figure 9.1. Pharmacy spirit award.

References

1. Purcell K. Pharmacy leadership survey: developing pharmacy leaders. *Texas Society of Health-System Pharmacists Journal.* 2004;5(2):8–15.

2. American Pharmaceutical Association Academy of Students of Pharmacy and American Association of Colleges of Pharmacy Council of Deans Task Force on Professionalism. White paper on pharmacy student professionalism. *J Am Pharm Assoc.* 2000;40:96–102.

3. Hammer DP, Berger BA, Beardsley RS, et al. Student professionalism. *Am J Pharm Educ.* 2003;67:Article 96.

4. American Board of Internal Medicine Committee on Evaluation of Clinical Competence and the Clinical Competence and Communication Programs. *Project Professionalism.* Philadelphia, PA: American Board of Internal Medicine; 2001:4–6.

5. Klein EJ, Jackson C, Kratz L, et al. Teaching professionalism to residents. *Acad Med.* 2003;78:26–34.

6. Accreditation Council for Pharmacy Education—Accreditation Standards and Guidelines 2007. Available at: http://www.acpe-accredit.org/standards/default.asp.

7. American Society of Health-System Pharmacists. ASHP statement on professionalism. *Am J Health Syst Pharm.* 2008;65:172–4.

8. Murphy JE. Confessions of a pharmacy thief. *Am J Health Syst Pharm.* 1996;53:2522–3.

9. White SJ. Career renewal. *Am J Health Syst Pharm.* 2008;65:119–21.

10. White SJ. Building and maintaining a professional network. *Am J Health Syst Pharm.* 2007;64:700–3.

11. White SJ, Tryon JE. How to find and succeed as a mentor. *Am J Health Syst Pharm.* 2007;64:1258–9.

12. Pascarella ER, Terenzini PT. *How College Affects Students: Findings and Insights from Twenty Years of Research.* San Francisco, CA: Jossey-Bass Publishers; 1991.

13. Kuh GD. The other curriculum: out-of-class experiences associated with student learning and personal development. *J Higher Educ.* 1995;66(2):123–55.

14. Miller TK, Jones JD. Out-of-class activities. In: Chickering AW, et al. *The Modern American College: Responding to the New Realities of Diverse Students and a Changing Society.* San Francisco, CA: Jossey-Bass Publishers; 1981:657–71.

15. Cox ER, Krueger KP, Murphy JE. Pharmacy student involvement in student organizations. *J Pharm Teaching.* 1998;6:9–18.

16. Harris RR, McConnell WE. The American Society of Hospital Pharmacists: a history. *Am J Hosp Pharm.* 1993;50(suppl 2):S1–S45.

17. ASHP Foundation website harveywhitney.org. *Whitney Award Lectures (1950–2007).* Bethesda, MD: ASHP Research and Education Foundation; 2007.

18. Worthen DB. Joseph Price Remington (1847–1918). *J Am Pharm Assoc.* 2002;42(4):664–6.

19. Emmons BF. Standing in the shadow of greatness. *Am J Health Syst Pharm.* 2008;65:360.

20. Peters, T. *The Brand You 50: Fifty Ways to Transform Yourself from an 'Employee' into a Brand That Shouts Distinction, Commitment, and Passion!* New York, NY: Alfred A. Knopf Inc; 1999.

21. Gazely B, Dignam M. *The Decision to Volunteer.* Washington, DC: ASAE & The Center for Association Leadership; 2008.

22. Purcell K. Pharmacy spirit. Catch it! Newsletter. *Texas Society of Health-System Pharmacists.* 1995;24(9):3,6.

23. Description of pharmacy spirit. Available at: http://www.tshp.org/About/Organizational Documents.asp. Accessed March 1, 2005.

What is the recipe for successful achievement? To my mind there are just four essential ingredients: Choose a career you love, give it the best there is in you, seize your opportunities, and be a member of the team.
Benjamin F. Fairless

Chapter 10

Career Advising

Michael D. Sanborn, Steven H. Dzierba, Dale E. English II, Bradi L. Frei, Darlene M. Mednick, Kevin Purcell, Jannet M. Carmichael, William N. Jones

Chapter Outline

Learning Objectives

- Describe ways in which preceptors can initially engage students in career planning discussions.
- Identify ways for preceptors and students to effectively participate in the career path planning process during and after rotations.
- Identify, contrast, and discuss the different career path opportunities available for pharmacists.
- Define, contrast, and provide general information on residencies and fellowships and their importance with respect to pharmacy practice.
- Discuss changes in the profession of pharmacy that may require additional training, education, and sound credentials based on clinical competencies.
- Describe other helpful methods to assist students in the career planning process.

Career advising is an important element of the preceptor-student interface. Preceptors have the ability to have an immeasurable impact on a student's career path and long-term job satisfaction. The enthusiastic preceptor who models professional pharmacy practice behavior and strives for excellence can ignite the student's passion for the profession. Oftentimes, the preceptor's interaction with a student is the first experience the student has had in that particular pharmacy environment. The doctor of pharmacy student that crosses the threshold of your pharmacy is not a blank slate but is a complex mixture of a multitude of life experiences that you may or may not share. However, preceptors will share this rotational experience with their students, and it is important to provide them with a positive and enlightening experience while introducing new career possibilities. For preceptors, helping students explore and plan different career paths is imperative regardless of the field or stage a preceptor or student is either entering or is currently in. The goal of this chapter is to assist the preceptor to expand and guide the student's knowledge regarding various pharmacy careers and the credentials needed to pursue them.

Pharmacy Practice Settings

Although it seems natural for a preceptor to guide students toward a particular career path relative to his or her own choices and views, avoid this, as students or residents should not overlook their unique characteristics and desires that contribute to their own career path. On the other hand, candid professional discussions regarding the pros and cons of all types of practice can be very helpful to students and can assist them with the difficult decision of what to do after graduation.

Many pharmacists traditionally begin their career in community- or hospital-based settings. Both settings have evolved to embrace pharmaceutical care in which pharmacists are directly responsible for achieving outcomes that improve a patient's quality of life. Also, pharmaceutical care now reaches across the continuum of care to allow pharmacists to be involved in everything from the development of clinical programs to decision-making for plan benefit programs administered by managed care organizations (MCOs), including pharmacy benefit managers (PBMs).

Pharmacist opportunities in healthcare continue to expand. Technology was once considered a threat but has ultimately lead to more career opportunities for pharmacists as seen in the increasing number of Internet pharmacies, the growth of electronic prescribing and electronic medical/health record (EMR/EHR) companies, and the evolution of the informatics pharmacist. Additionally, when the Medicare prescription benefit was implemented it provided many opportunities for pharmacists to help beneficiaries understand their benefit, the concepts of a medication formulary, and become more involved in medication therapy management (MTM).

A preceptor can tailor the rotational experience to facilitate career planning in two ways. The first way is to tailor the experience to the student's interests and to expand the student's knowledge base of those areas while continuously pointing out career paths that match student interest. Conversely, the rotation can cover gaps in the students' knowledge with exposure to new practice environments (such as introduction to an HIV clinic, leadership opportunities, or investigational drug service) and may expand the student's existing knowledge to career paths that would have otherwise been unknown. The route your rotation will take is a decision you, as a preceptor, must make, which means that it may not always be exactly what the student wants or initially expects.

Career Planning: The Preceptor's Role

A preceptor's role is not only to help the student learn, but also to integrate those learning experiences into a foundation for a successful career. As discussed, a good preceptor will see part of his or her role as an opportunity to introduce students to new professional encounters that expand their understanding of the breadth and depth of pharmacy practice.

The first step in assisting the student with their career planning process is to assess the student's understanding of the pharmacy field and career goals. Discovering which pharmacy environments the student has experienced can help; the student may be overlooking certain career opportunities because he or she has decided that a certain area is not a good fit, even though he or she may not have any direct experience in that particular practice specialty. In this situation, it is helpful to initiate an open discussion focusing on tailoring the rotation to fit career goals and providing the student with possible unique rotation options. After reviewing the available options, allow the student to reflect on these options and formulate a thoughtful response. Although it may feel uncomfortable, this active listening process is important and will give the student time to weigh the options and respond with complete, intelligent responses. The key is to listen. Be a sounding board for the student, who may rarely have the opportunity to share his or her ideas and plans with an experienced pharmacist.

• Preceptor Pearls •

Start a conversation with the student about career planning. Consider using the following:

- What are your plans after pharmacy school?
- What areas of pharmacy practice did you find most interesting?
- What did you like doing the most on your rotations?
- What tasks or responsibilities in pharmacy do you get the most praise for?
- What are the important things to you in relation to a pharmacy career (i.e., money, praise, challenge, fame)?
- Describe a project or task you really enjoyed.
- Are there areas of pharmacy practice to which you have not been exposed?

Always provide students with feedback regarding their ideas about their career path and planning in a timely, constructive, and positive manner. Throughout the rotation, preceptors can discuss and review various rotation experiences as they relate to career options. Effective methods of impacting the student's career choices include the following:

- Discuss alternative career options that the student may not have considered.
- Expose the student to additional experiences within his or her desired area of practice.
- Review career path enhancements such as residencies and fellowships.
- Continuously coach students regarding next steps as they move towards a desired career path.
- Review career resources that are available to the student.

An important part of career exposure requires the student to develop a potential network of professional contacts. The preceptor can be invaluable in assisting with this effort. It is important to encourage the student to develop a critical appraisal of possible career options. Have the student begin to identify the advantages and disadvantages of various career options from his or her point of view. Also remember that, while you may find a particular aspect of a career as a positive, your student may find it as a negative. For example, some students may initially be intimidated by rounding with physicians and other healthcare professionals as part of the healthcare team. Work with the student to build confidence in this role, but also understand that it may be something that they do not truly enjoy.

It is also helpful to review your own career path and share your experiences—both positive and negative—and discuss why you have made the career decisions that you have made. A good mentor should share these personal and professional experiences and provide examples of areas of career success and opportunities for improvement. Engage students in asking why things did or did not work. Every preceptor has lived through situations that could be useful if shared with an engaged student.

Career Planning: Generating Interest Among Students

There are some unique ways to increase the student's interest and participation in career planning. Preceptors can help students start their career planning efforts by asking them to visualize the end of their careers. Some mentors may ask students for their 5- or 10-year plans, or use another unique method, which may include asking the student to develop an obituary, a life purpose statement, or principles of practice statement. Fred Eckel, a pharmacy professor at the University of North Carolina, has assisted many health-system leaders using this future reflection process. Students who participate in this type of activity often walk away with a detailed career plan that they believe in. They can then begin to implement and revise this plan throughout their lives. Decision-making becomes clearer and easier when they have a more detailed vision of the future.

Another way for preceptors to generate interest in career planning is to encourage the student to become involved in professional organizations outside of work. This is an important way for students to develop a professional network, to expose themselves to expanded career opportunities, and to gain experience. Working in local, state, and national organizations will also help develop skills needed for future roles. Students need exposure to as many of the potential opportunities that will be available to them in the future.[1]

Careers in Pharmacy

Diverse career opportunities available today signify a robust opportunity for pharmacists to choose thoughtfully between practice settings, taking into consideration their unique talents, interests, skills, and competencies, along with balancing personal and professional life. The variety of choices today, versus the more historical and limited choices of the past, has created greater challenges for practicing professionals (and employers of pharmacists) to create work environments that understand and reflect both educational achievement and growing generational diversity.

Many pharmacists have sought practice settings that more fully utilize their skills and abilities yet also allow for growth in their careers. Pharmacists have many opportunities well beyond the more traditional product-based dispensing, distribution, supervision of technicians, and delivery of medications. Many pharmacists have sought practice settings that more fully utilize their skills and allow for growth in their careers. These settings present pharmacists with almost limitless opportunities to impact patient care. In fact many of these newer nontraditional practice settings have been the driving force behind the changing roles seen today.

Although it is true that diverse practice settings and career opportunities for pharmacists have never been greater, it is the remarkable advancement of the profession that allows for highly talented and motivated pharmacists to exist at many important points along the healthcare continuum. Thus, it is even more important now that faculty, preceptors, mentors, and residency program directors be as familiar as possible with these opportunities to provide guidance to students and to provide for a match between skills, competencies, and personal objectives.

As a preceptor, students will look to you for insight concerning possible pharmacy career opportunities. It is important for you to have some background on many of the different pharmacy career options, and it may be possible for you to assist the student in learning more about a particular type of practice. It is also important for you to be aware of each student's strengths as well as weaknesses and what role these may play in their future pharmacy career options. Your particular insight about pharmacy careers should stimulate the student to further investigate on their own what may be best for them knowing this will likely change based on multiple contributing factors in their lifetime.

As a preceptor you may be able to utilize your own network of colleagues if necessary. You may assist the student in making a connection with a colleague in a particular pharmacy practice setting to allow the student greater insight into that career option. It is important to note that as preceptors we should allow our enthusiasm for the profession to engulf the student and to be supportive of their pharmacy career choice, whatever that may be.

It is impossible to develop a comprehensive outline of all current practice settings available to pharmacists, and the opportunities will continue to expand given the ever-changing healthcare system in the U.S. This is a positive testament to the flexibility of the profession. The following information outlines many of the current, broader practice settings available to pharmacists, and covers the expanding opportunities relative to the changing healthcare system in the U.S.

Box 10.1 summarizes some of the many examples of careers currently available to pharmacists. In almost all of these settings, pharmacists collaborate with physicians, nurses, administrators, and other healthcare professionals to develop, implement, and monitor a therapeutic plan that ensures satisfactory clinical, economic, and humanistic outcomes for the patient. A detailed discussion of some of the more common types of practice setting follows, and sharing this information with a student can be quite valuable as they continue to develop their own career path.

Box 10.1 • List of Common Career Opportunities for Pharmacists

Community pharmacy

Compounding

Institutional (health-system) pharmacy

Drug information

Home care/LTC (long-term care) pharmacy

Managed care pharmacy

Pharmaceutical industry

Regulatory affairs

Academia

Research

Consultant pharmacy

Government practice

Civic and political leadership

Box 10.1. List of Common Career Opportunities for Pharmacists (cont'd)

Military service

Nuclear pharmacy

Nutrition support

Clinical specialist (oncology, infectious disease, cardiology, etc.)

Operating room pharmacist

Pediatric pharmacist

Poison control

Veterinary pharmacist

Professional associations

Employee benefit consulting

Clinical research organizations (CROs)

Medical marketing and communication organizations

Pharmaceutical and healthcare distributors

Healthcare information technology

Emergency department pharmacist

Medication safety officer

Community Pharmacy

Community practice is probably the most familiar type of pharmacy practice to the American public. It employs a large number of pharmacists—in fact six out of 10 pharmacists provide care to patients in a community setting.[2] Pharmacists in a community setting provide information and advice on health, provide medications and associated services, and refer patients to other sources of help and care when necessary. Many community pharmacies have developed further specialties in durable medical equipment (DME), homeopathic medicine, and customized compounding.

Community pharmacists also assist patients in understanding their prescription benefit program and may provide disease and care management in a variety of areas, including diabetes, asthma, hypertension, and hyperlipidemia. Many pharmacists achieve specialty certifications in these key disease areas in order to better educate and assist patients in managing their healthcare. Unfortunately, many community pharmacy practice settings have continued to use pharmacists in a more traditional dispensing role rather than fit these other activities into their operational and business model.

Significant management and entrepreneurial opportunities also exist for those with interest and abilities in this area. Supervising a retail store, owning or operating a private compounding pharmacy, or serving as a district manager for a large retail chain are examples of such leadership opportunities. Although many of the skills and competencies required for such roles can be achieved through experience or on-the-job training, additional instruction in areas of business, process engineering, quality tools, and leadership can be valuable in achieving these types of positions.

Institutional (Health-System) Pharmacy

There has been an increased need for pharmacists to provide care through organized healthcare settings, including hospitals, nursing homes, extended care facilities, neighborhood health centers, and ambulatory care clinics. While pharmacists work in these settings as drug information experts and systems control experts, they are also responsible for controlling drug distribution and systems to ensure that patients receive the appropriate medications. Many pharmacists are involved in pharmacy and therapeutics (P&T) committees as well as preparing drug monographs and therapeutic class reviews. Performance improvement activities such as developing and performing drug utilization review (DUR) programs, as well as educating other healthcare professionals within the organization, are yet another large component of a hospital pharmacist's role and responsibilities.

The focus on medical errors revealed by the Institute of Medicine reports, *To Err is Human: Building a Safer Health System* and *Preventing Medication Errors: Quality Chasm Series*, has enabled pharmacists who have a systems aptitude to become involved in organization- or enterprise-wide teams and to be primary participants in teams that are working to implement complex safety systems such as computerized physician order entry (CPOE), bedside bar-code scanning, and other decision support technology within automated systems.

Pharmacists in health systems typically work with physicians and nurses in a collaborative team environment to provide direct patient care. These roles require pharmacists to possess additional competencies such as excellent communication skills, influence and persuasion, capabilities, negotiation skills, and critical-thinking/problem-solving skills.

Box 10.2 identifies some of the unique areas in which pharmacists in institutional practice as well as other practice settings specialize. Note that these areas often require additional training such as a specialty residency and/or board certification.

Box 10.2 • Areas of Specialization

Nuclear pharmacy
Infectious diseases
Psychiatry
Nutrition
Oncology
Internal medicine
Cardiology
Drug information
Nephrology
Geriatrics
Critical care pharmacy
Pediatrics
Poison control
Primary care
ER medicine

Many pharmacists also pursue leadership positions within health-system practice, in which there are a variety of opportunities available. Management of clinical services, patient care operations, and department technology also offer rewarding career paths and opportunities for advancement. Administrative positions at the director or chief pharmacy officer level offer an even more expansive level of responsibility in the areas of finance, drug use policy, personnel management, and setting the department's overall direction. These positions may also require additional educational training, such as a specialized administrative residency combined with a master's degree.

Long-Term Care Pharmacy

Pharmacists practicing in long-term care practice settings are responsible for drug information, education, and drug therapy management of a growing segment of our population. This area of pharmacy is practiced in home care agencies, adult day-care centers, hospices, and other long-term care facilities.

These patients often require DUR and adjustments to drug therapy due to diminished hepatic and renal functions, and to the quantity of medications this population often uses. Given the increased medication use and longer life expectancies, along with the "baby-boomer" population accessing more health services, specialization in geriatric pharmacy is expected to grow rapidly.

Managed Care Pharmacy

Managed care pharmacy practice has grown dramatically within the last decade due to the need to manage the increase in healthcare expenditures, especially the double-digit trend in drug costs. Providing a prescription drug program as a part of the medical benefit has become increasingly difficult for many employers and other payers who recognize the importance of providing access to prescription drugs.

Many payers (government, employers, etc.) contract MCOs, including health plans and PBMs, to help manage the quality, cost, and access of a prescription drug benefit. The primary goal is to ensure that what is spent on prescription drugs is appropriate and safe, as well as to ensure that medications are properly used. There are thousands of pharmacists practicing in a managed care setting.[3]

Managed care pharmacists are responsible for plan design; clinical program development; clinical management; pharmacoeconomic analysis; outcomes research; communication and education of patients, prescribers, and pharmacists; and drug distribution and dispensing, as well as performing the clinical interventions to support the DUR, formulary management, and disease management of the populations that MCO serves. Pharmacists are also more and more involved in the development, administration, and management of the pharmacy provider networks that provide care to patients, as well as in the performance and quality monitoring, reporting, auditing, and contracting of the network and services.

Another area within a health plan or PBM where a pharmacist's unique skills are valued is in the pharmaceutical contracting group. There, pharmacists monitor manufacturers' drug pipelines and develop forecasting models to determine the impact of that drug on a payer's program. In addition, they are often responsible for clinically assessing and evaluating the product, negotiating the purchase or use of contracts, developing and implementing the programs designed to maximize the formulary, and recommending formulary decisions and administration.

Several large employers and insurers have also recognized the value and expertise of pharmacists in designing and managing a benefit and have hired pharmacists as a part of their managed medical team, many taking on roles of chief pharmacy officer (CPO)—similar to the CMO (chief medical officer)—within the management team. The integration of pharmacy into the medical strategy is very important in achieving the goals of quality, cost management, and access.

Many MCOs use mail order or online services as a management tool within the benefit. This creates opportunities for pharmacists as managers of operations (pharmacies owned and operated by the MCO or contracted entities), as well as specialists in key areas like targeted DUR programs, formulary management (including generic and therapeutic substitution), and disease management programs.

Specialty Pharmacy

Managing biotechnology and self-administered injectables is a growing area of concern for many MCOs and pharmaceutical manufacturers due to the complexity of the drug administration need for specific patient education/management, and unique product storage requirements. Further, the cost of these drugs is usually high and, therefore, ensuring proper use, administration, storage, and management is important.

Until recently these self-administered drugs have often been paid for as part of the medical benefit and have not been managed as unique products requiring additional services. There is a growing trend to "carve out" the management of these drug products usually through the PBM or health plan. As a result, there are more specialty pharmacy organizations that focus only on the management of these drug therapies. The growth is directly related to the required, related services due to the complexity of therapy and the need for patient education, as well as to the growing number of biotechnology drugs available to treat diseases.

This provides pharmacists with another area of specialty practice focused on supporting patients living with complex health conditions. This includes education on the storage, administration, and special handling and delivery requirements for these products. See Box 10.3 for examples of complicated diseases in which pharmacists play a critical role in clinical program development.

With the growing number of biotechnology products available and/or expected and the advent of pharmacogenomics, this is certainly an exciting time for pharmacists who want to pursue this field to utilize their clinical and business management skills.

Box 10.3 • Complicated Diseases for Pharmacists

Acromegaly	Chronic granulomatous disease
Cystic fibrosis	Gaucher disease
Growth hormone disorders	Viral hepatitis
HIV/AIDS	Infertility
Multiple sclerosis	Oncology-related conditions
Psoriasis	Rheumatoid arthritis
Solid organ transplant	

Pharmaceutical Industry

The pharmaceutical industry provides many career opportunities for pharmacists. It is not only broad in its offerings, but it continues to evolve. In this industry, pharmacists hold positions in sales, training and education, clinical research, product development, marketing, outcomes research, pharmacoeconomics, regulatory affairs, epidemiology, clinical trials, and administration. Many pharmacists involved in pharmaceutical companies go on to obtain postgraduate degrees in order to meet the technical demands and scientific duties required in pharmaceutical manufacturing and general business management.[2]

Pharmacists with an interest in sales and administration can combine their clinical expertise in positions such as medical service representatives or liaisons, or clinical educators. Like many other areas of practice, the roles for pharmacists have grown tremendously; however, industry pharmacists typically do not have patient contact.

Another growth opportunity within the pharmaceutical industry is the medical information group, which is responsible for off-label drug information questions and the preparation of the product dossier that is a required part of the Format for Formulary Submission.[3] Additional opportunities exist in generic drug companies as well as in wholesale drug companies.

Academia and Research

Another rewarding career opportunity for pharmacists is serving in either a part- or full-time capacity within a college of pharmacy. In this role, pharmacists are responsible for the teaching and education of the future members of the profession. Many faculty members hold administrative and management positions within the university or college, or they teach in other health sciences areas. They are also involved in research; public service; and consulting to local, state, national, and international organizations. Becoming a member of the faculty at a college of pharmacy may require a postgraduate degree and/or training (e.g., Ph.D., or residency or fellowship training following the professional degree program).

In addition to teaching and research, many pharmacy practice faculty have active patient care responsibilities and precept students during internships and clerkships (experiential rotations). Pharmacists can also hold faculty positions in pharmaceutical sciences research, in which an expertise in study design, methodology, and analytics is required to solve complex problems of drug utilization management healthcare delivery, marketing, management, and other practice issues.[2] It has been stated that "Perhaps no other job in pharmacy has such far-reaching effects on the profession as that of an educator. It is in academia that one can excite individuals about pharmacy and lay the groundwork for continuing advances in the field."[2]

Consultant Pharmacy

Consultant pharmacists provide expert advice on the use of medications by individuals or within institutions, or on the provision of pharmacy services to institutions. The phrase "consultant pharmacist," coined by George F. Archambault, who is considered the founding father of consultant pharmacy, originated in the nursing home environment when a group of innovative pharmacists focused on improving the use of medications in these facilities. However, consultant pharmacists are found today in a variety of other settings, including subacute care and assisted-living facilities, psychiatric hospitals, hospice programs, and in-home and community-based care.[4]

In addition to the more traditional definition and description above, there are increasing numbers of experienced pharmacists who consult in a variety of areas of expertise from managed care, to specialty disease areas or populations, to electronic prescribing and plan design. Many pharmacists work for individual consulting companies providing expertise and advice associated with different areas of pharmacy practice and healthcare management.

Government

Traditionally pharmacists can be employed in staff and supervisory positions by the government at the Federal level, in the Departments of Public Health Service, the Veterans Administration, the Food and Drug Administration, and the Armed Services. At the state and local levels they are employed by regulatory, health, and social service agencies, including agencies charged with regulating the practice of pharmacy to preserve and protect the public health. As some state health agencies are consolidating their purchases, pharmacists are also engaged in procuring supplies for the entire state. Some positions provide commissioned officer status whereas others are under civil service. Other pharmacists hold positions within state Medicaid programs, especially in the DUR boards formed by many states.

Additional important and exciting opportunities are beginning to take shape due to the passage of the Medicare Prescription Drug, Improvement, and Modernization Act (MMA) of 2003. Already there are several pharmacists who have been hired at Centers for Medicare and Medicaid Services (CMS) and who have served as experts and committee leaders in organizations such as the National Committee on Vital and Health Statistics (NCVHS) and the National Quality Forum (NQF). Finally, there are some pharmacists who have been elected to political office at the local, state, and national levels.

Professional Associations

Pharmacists also have careers in state and national professional associations. Several national professional associations are led and staffed by pharmacists with an interest and special talent in organizational work, including educational programming and services, meeting planning and management, writing, project management, research, and fundraising.

Below are some of the largest and most well-known pharmacy practice associations:

- ASHP—American Society of Health-System Pharmacists
- APhA—American Pharmacists Association
- AMCP—Academy of Managed Care Pharmacy
- ASCP—American Society of Consultant Pharmacists
- ACCP—American College of Clinical Pharmacy
- FIP—International Pharmaceutical Federation

These organizations represent large groups of pharmacists and are instrumental in shaping practice trends. Their advocacy role for the profession is also critically important.

Employee Benefit Consulting

As mentioned in the managed care section, payers are facing a significant challenge in providing a healthcare benefit, and there is an increased focus on the prescription drug program. Typically payers do not have the clinical expertise in-house and have been using benefit consultants (e.g., Mercer, AON, etc.) to help with plan design and benefit management, as well as their expertise and knowledge in selecting a PBM. Many even continue to use these organizations to manage the PBM relationship. Pharmacists with managed care and business experience are finding rewarding careers in these benefit consultant organizations as clinical program managers, account or client service managers, and as in-house experts in developing and reviewing PBM services and contracts.

Contract Research Organizations

Contract research organizations (CROs) design, manage, monitor, and analyze preclinical and clinical trials. These services are provided to the pharmaceutical industry and are increasingly valuable because the clinical trials are the bases for determining the safety and efficacy of pharmaceuticals, biologics, and medical devices. These organizations have experienced increased popularity and growth over the last several years as the rigor and complexity of medication research increases. CROs will continue to provide career opportunities for pharmacists, especially in the Phase IV clinical trials now required by the FDA.

Medical Marketing and Communication Organizations

Many pharmacists who excel at written and verbal communication skills have found exciting careers at medical communications companies, which develop clinical content for educational and promotional programs and publications for clinical and management professionals. Positions can be either staff or supervisory and typically focus on the following areas; medical writing, program development, project management, clinical education, meeting planning and management, strategy, facilitation, business development, and account management.

Pharmaceutical and Healthcare Distributors

Distributors are an essential part of the pharmaceutical supply chain, and their chief role is to simplify and consolidate the purchasing process. Pharmacists in these organization ensure that the medications and other healthcare products needed to diagnose, prevent, and treat illnesses are distributed to the appropriate locations. In addition to the delivery of these products, many pharmaceutical and healthcare distributors have expanded their service offerings to include information management, automation, program development, consulting, and other tools to improve their customer's efficiency and effectiveness.

Pharmacists play a valuable role in all of these expanded services from designing and developing the programs, to the implementation and delivery of them. An important function of pharmaceutical and healthcare distributors is protecting the quality and security of the products distributed. They also provide economies of scale to reduce distribution expenses, manage inventories to ensure product availability, and simplify distribution to ensure vital medication is available where and when it is needed.

Group Purchasing Organizations

Group purchasing organizations (GPOs) primarily provide contracting services to hospitals, clinics, and health systems. Pharmacists employed in this area assist with contract management and vendor evaluation for pharmaceuticals and other products, and may also be involved in the development and provision of other services such as monograph development, data analysis, education, and consulting.

Healthcare Information Technology Companies

Many students and new practitioners are familiar and comfortable with healthcare technology. In fact, many use online resources more frequently than any other resource, often using the Internet and company websites over more traditional sources of information. Therefore, it stands to reason that many are interested in careers that combine technical pharmacy knowledge with technology to deliver more integrated, efficient, and safe healthcare. In addition to healthcare information technology companies, a growing number of electronic prescribing companies, offering EMRs and EHRs, employ pharmacists as domain experts or in program development and management.

The goal of the healthcare industry is to enhance patient safety by accelerating the adoption of information technology. This is especially evident in the new MMA provisions on e-prescribing and in the president's mandate for electronic health records for all Americans by 2015. Pharmacists can play a significant role in helping to design, develop, and implement prescribing standards within information technology companies. They can also play an important role in bringing together healthcare providers and professionals in achieving this goal.

Advanced Pharmacy Training

As the complexity of pharmacy practice continues to grow, advanced postgraduate training becomes increasingly important. Graduating with a doctor of pharmacy degree provides pharmacists with a broad scope of knowledge in a variety of settings. However, practicing pharmacists— especially those in direct patient care roles—often need to attain advanced practice knowledge and enhance their clinical skills. Pharmacists are charged with both professional and legal responsibility for all medication-use activities. That responsibility is clear in professional standards, statutes, regulations, and external quality standards. In addition, the complexity of medication ingredients and products will continue to expand.

Pharmacy Residencies

In preparing themselves for future opportunities and leadership positions, students should consider completing a pharmacy residency. The American College of Clinical Pharmacy (ACCP) and the American Society of Health-System Pharmacists (ASHP) have both adopted positions whereby pharmacists will be expected to complete residency training if they will provide direct patient care.[5,6]

Increasingly, employers are also seeking pharmacists who have completed an accredited residency. Completing a residency is also important to the development of clinical maturity. Pharmacy graduates may have a broad scope of knowledge, but they may not have the confidence to apply that knowledge to optimize drug therapy for their patients. A pharmacy residency gives residents the opportunity to enhance their confidence and sharpen their skills in assuring that patients are receiving the best care possible. As stated, pharmacists who aspire to an academic career will be expected to have residency training as a minimum requirement.[7]

Pharmacy residencies are critical in producing clinicians, managers, and leaders for the pharmacy profession. The role of residency training has been heightened by changes in the delivery of healthcare and in the opportunities that are being afforded to pharmacists for drug therapy management and for health promotion and disease prevention activities. Healthcare reimbursement changes have resulted in a redistribution of patient care from the inpatient to the outpatient setting, which has increased the acuity level of patients in both settings. Pharmacists with more specialized knowledge and training are needed to manage these very complex patients. Beyond more practice complexity is the move toward the use of much higher technology processing.

New standards for residency programs were released in 2005, and fully implemented in 2007.[8] The major change in the standards was modifying the terminology to postgraduate year-one (PGY1) and postgraduate year-two (PGY2).[9] Residencies are no longer classified as general, pharmacy practice, or specialized pharmacy residencies. The specific definitions of PGY1 and PGY2 residencies are listed in Box 10.4.

Box 10.4 • Summary Explanation of Residency Types

Postgraduate Year One (PGY1) Residency

Postgraduate year one of pharmacy residency training is an organized, directed, accredited program that builds on knowledge, skills, attitudes, and abilities gained from an accredited professional pharmacy degree program. The first-year residency program enhances general competencies in managing medication-use systems and supports optimal medication therapy outcomes for patients with a broad range of disease states.

Postgraduate Year Two (PGY2) Residency

Postgraduate year two of pharmacy residency training is an organized, directed, accredited program that builds on the competencies established in postgraduate year one of residency training. The second-year residency program is focused in a specific area of practice. The PGY2 program increases the resident's depth of knowledge, skills, attitudes, and abilities to raise the resident's level of expertise in medication therapy management and clinical leadership in the area of focus. In those practice areas where board certification exists, graduates are prepared to pursue such certification.[4]

Pharmacy Fellowships

Another postgraduate training route is pharmacy fellowship. Unlike a residency, fellowships are designed to prepare the participant in becoming an independent researcher. Fellowships are typically 2 years in duration, and based in pharmacy schools or academic health centers. The ACCP defines fellowships as a minimum of 3,000 hours over 2 years that is devoted to research activities. ACCP lists 21 different categories for fellowship training in 62 different locations in 2008.[10] There is also a voluntary peer review process among these fellowship programs aimed at improving the preceptors and research programs. See Box 10.5 for additional resources on residencies and fellowships.

Box 10.5 • Resources on Residencies and Fellowships

Residencies:

- Visit the ASHP website (www.ashp.org). The site includes definitions, accreditation standards, a directory of accredited programs, the resident matching program, the residency showcase, links to the regional residency conference websites, and federal funding.
- Managed care pharmacy residencies: Visit the AMCP website (www.amcp.org).
- Community pharmacy residencies: Visit the APhA website (www.aphanet.org).

Fellowships:

- Visit the ACCP website (www.accp.com). The site includes a listing of fellowships and residencies.

The Case for Additional Credentials

Students with both short- and long-term career plans should consider the types of education, training, and credentials that will be required or helpful to help position them for desired future opportunities. Professional growth and development, lifelong learning, and career advancement necessitate continuous pursuit of new knowledge and skills. This may go beyond what is acquired through attending routine continuing education programs and engaging in self-directed, independent study. Medical and pharmaceutical information is increasing at an exponential rate. The practice of pharmacy is changing and adapting based on new professional needs. Fortunately, there are many options available for working pharmacists to obtain additional education, training, and credentials, including focused education courses, advanced degrees, skills-based training workshops, and certifications.

The long-range vision or strategic plan for pharmacy practice shows that much has been written about the need for the profession to become "clinical." What this means broadly is that most pharmacists of the future are expected to be clinical pharmacy practitioners who provide advanced patient care services. This consensus represents the opinion of multiple pharmacy organizations with the shared vision that "pharmacists will be the healthcare professionals responsible for providing patient care that ensures optimal medication therapy outcomes."[11] The Joint Commission of Pharmacy Practitioners (JCPP) vision for 2015 is pharmacy that education will prepare a pharmacist to provide patient-centered and population-based care.

Advanced Education

Focused education courses are typically offered by a university or by a university working in partnership with a professional society or healthcare organization (employer). The most visible examples are executive management and leadership courses. These vary in length from intensive weeklong courses to full semester courses delivered during the evenings or on the weekends. This option may be good for pharmacists who want education in a specific area but do not want to invest the time, money, and effort into completing an entire degree program. The week-long courses do not provide college credit, but the full semester courses usually do, and this credit may possibly be applied to obtaining a degree in the future.

Master's and doctoral degree programs are offered in a variety of fields that may be of benefit to practicing pharmacists, and many universities have master's and doctoral degree programs targeted toward working adults. These can be distance education programs provided either online or through a variety of media or campus-based programs offered during the evenings or on the weekends. Pharmacists commonly obtain master's degrees in hospital pharmacy administration (MS), business administration (MBA), healthcare administration (MHA), and public health (MPH). These credentials may be important when pursuing administrative positions in hospitals and other healthcare organizations.

Some pharmacists may even decide to obtain a doctoral degree in one of these areas (e.g., Ph.D., DBA, DHA, or Dr.PH.), especially if they work in an academic health center and are heavily involved in teaching students, residents, and fellows. Some pharmacists whose primary responsibility is teaching obtain a master's degree (M.Ed.) or a doctoral degree (Ph.D.) in education. This is particularly useful in academia when the pharmacist is responsible for curriculum development and outcomes assessment, faculty development, distance education programs, and experiential education programs. Of course, many pharmacists have obtained a nontraditional doctor of pharmacy degree. These programs have been important for pharmacists transitioning from a drug distribution role to a patient care role. Finally, a few pharmacists go back to graduate school full-time to obtain a doctoral degree in one of the pharmaceutical sciences (Ph.D.) and pursue a research-oriented career track in academia or the pharmaceutical industry. Keep in mind that some employers may pay for their employees to complete master's or doctoral programs if it will better prepare them for their current position or for a future position with the organization.

Skills-based workshops are offered in a variety of clinical areas (e.g., basic clinical skills, physical assessment, anticoagulation, asthma, diabetes, immunizations, and herbals). Skills-based workshops are usually developed by pharmacy professional organizations and pharmacy schools. These skills-based workshops are typically one or two days in length and provide continuing education approved by the Accreditation Council for Pharmacy Education (ACPE). Some of these workshops are linked to certification programs. This option may be good for pharmacists who want focused training in a specific area, especially those looking to expand the scope of their practice. Also, various healthcare organizations offer skills-based certification courses in basic cardiac life support (BCLS) and advanced cardiac life support (ACLS). These can be useful for anyone in general, especially BCLS, and they are of particular importance in institutions where pharmacists serve as members of the code team.

Competencies and Credentials

A credential is simply any formally documented evidence of qualifications. The credentials needed to enter pharmacy practice for new practitioners include

- Graduation from an Accreditation Council for Pharmacy Education (ACPE) accredited Pharm.D. training program
- Successfully passing the National Association of Boards of Pharmacy License Examination (NABPLEX)

- Fulfillment of any additional state board of pharmacy licensure requirements (e.g., state law exam, internship hours, etc.)

Pharmacists with the above credentials can independently and legally provide patient care and manage pharmacotherapy. However, a pharmacist may seek further credentials when comparing the different competencies that must be met by a recent pharmacy graduate with those of pharmacists having more training and experience.

Pharmacists develop proficiency through both formal training and practice experience. For example, during doctor of pharmacy degree training programs, students are exposed to broad disease state training and experiences promoting general therapeutic principles. Competency statements are written by each college of pharmacy for all aspects of training and education. ACPE doctor of pharmacy accreditation curricular standards state that "graduates must possess the basic knowledge, skills, and abilities to practice pharmacy independently, at the time of graduation."[12]

There are a variety of credentials that pharmacists voluntarily earn to document their advanced or specialized knowledge and skills.[13] These credentials are earned when pharmacists complete competencies that are beyond those earned in doctor of pharmacy programs. As discussed, postgraduate year one (PGY1) residency programs are designed around competency statements that offer the pharmacist additional training beyond those learned in Pharm.D. programs and deepen a pharmacist's knowledge as well as promote the development of better patient care skills, problem solving and clinical judgment. Although preferred, PGY1 residencies are not the only way to develop this higher level of knowledge, skill and ability, but are probably the shortest way to achieving the desired competencies. In addition, when residency programs are accredited by a national accrediting body such as the Commission on Credentialing of ASHP, others in the profession can be assured programs and graduates will meet certain minimum standards.

We have also learned that postgraduate year two (PGY2) residency programs allow residents to develop even more in-depth knowledge and skills by working in specialized or differentiated areas of practice. Educators tell us that repetition is essential in the development of any practice skill; therefore, the level of performance of a pharmacist depends on the amount of patient care practice time devoted to develop that skill. Developing the skills "correctly" can most effectively be done under the supervision of another skilled practitioner who can prepare and mentor the learner for more complex problem solving, decision making, and independence. While meeting competency statements assigned through educational programs or attaining credentials does not assure a practitioner's competence to practice, a key factor in developing competence is the continual learning of new knowledge and the enhancement of critical thinking and problem solving skills through practice.

Quality Assurance and Improvement

Many efforts are underway to improve the quality of healthcare in the U.S. Activities that contribute to defining, assessing, monitoring and improving the quality of patient care are referred to as *quality assurance*.[14] *Quality improvement* is a method of planning and implementing continuous improvements in systems or processes in order to provide quality healthcare reflected by improved patient outcomes. Credentials of healthcare providers are used by healthcare quality assurance organizations such as The Joint Commission (TJC) and the National Committee for Quality Assurance (NCQA) as indicators of competence and qualifications to provide certain levels of patient care service. These organizations are promoting rules that determine which providers can provide certain types of services to provide the highest levels of patient care.[15]

Credentialing is the process by which an organization or institution obtains, verifies and assesses a pharmacist's qualifications to provide patient care services.[16] Credentialing and Privileging are determined by the bylaws or policies of a healthcare organization. Credentialing is required for many types of healthcare professionals to be hired in a health system and determines their level of specific patient care services.[15] As discussed, credentials in the pharmacy profession can be obtained through a variety of mechanisms. For example, in addition to the credentials that we have already listed pharmacists may complete a lengthy and targeted disease state-education program or become board certified.

Certification programs are defined by ACPE as "structured and systematic postgraduate continuing education experiences for pharmacists that are generally smaller in magnitude and shorter in time than degree programs, and that impart knowledge, skills, attitudes, and performance behaviors designed to meet specific pharmacy practice objectives."[17] Certification programs should not be confused with continuing education (CE) which is needed in most states for relicensure. Compared to CE, certification programs are designed to expand practice competencies, usually in a specific area (e.g., smoking cessation, diabetes education, immunization, and anticoagulation).

Pharmacy Board Certification

Certification is a voluntary process by which a nongovernmental agency or an association grants recognition to an individual who has met certain predetermined qualifications specified by that organization. This formal recognition is granted to designate to the public that the individual has attained the requisite level of knowledge, skill, and/or experience in a well-defined, often specialized, area of the total discipline. Certification usually requires initial assessment and periodic reassessments of the individual's knowledge, skills, and/or experience. Certification can be a useful credential for pharmacists in either a clinical or a management career track.

Certification is a credential granted to pharmacists and other health professionals who have demonstrated a level of competence in a specific and relatively narrow area of practice that exceeds the minimum requirements for licensure. Certification is granted on the basis of successful completion of rigorously developed eligibility criteria that include a written examination and, in some cases, an experiential component. The certification process for pharmacy is undertaken and overseen by the Board of Pharmaceutical Specialties (BPS) or the Commission on Certification in Geriatric Pharmacy (CCGP).

The development of a certification program includes the following steps:

1. Defining the area in which certification is offered (role delineation)

2. Creating and administering a psychometrically valid content-based examination

3. Identifying other criteria for awarding the credential (e.g., experience)

4. Identifying recertification criteria[17]

A breakout of each of these steps is outlined below:

• Role delineation. The first step is to define the area in which certification is to be offered.

This is done through a process called role delineation or "task analysis." An expert panel of individuals in the proposed subject area develops a survey instrument to assess how practitioners working in the area rate the importance, frequency, and criticality of specific activities in that practice. The instrument is then sent to a sample of pharmacists who are practicing in that field.

- Development of content outline. On the basis of responses to the survey, a content outline for the certification program is developed.

- Preparation of examination. The written examination component of the certification program is developed on the basis of the content outline.

- Other activities. Appropriate measures are taken to ensure that security and confidentially of the testing process are maintained, that the examination and eligibility criteria are appropriate, and that the knowledge and skills of those who are certified do, in fact, reflect competence.

In 1976 the American Pharmaceutical Association (APhA) established the BPS to grant specialty certification to qualified pharmacists. Since that time five specialties share the BPS core mission which is to improve patient care through recognition and promotion of high level training, knowledge, and skills in pharmacy through board certification of pharmacists.[18] BPS certifies pharmacists in five specialty areas and the American Society of Consultant Pharmacists (ASCP) oversees a certification program in geriatric pharmacy practice listed in Box 10.6. In addition to specialty certification, BPS will provide "added qualification" within the pharmacotherapy specialty for enhanced level of training and experience within cardiology or infectious diseases.

Box 10.6 • Currently Recognized Pharmacy Board Specialties

Pharmacotherapy

Includes two added qualifications in infectious diseases and cardiology) and is designated board-certified pharmacotherapy specialists (BCPS)

Nuclear Pharmacy

Designated board-certified nuclear pharmacists (BCNP)

Nutrition Support Pharmacy

Designated board-certified nutrition support pharmacists (BCNSP)

Psychiatric Pharmacy Practice

Designated board-certified psychiatric pharmacists (BCPP)

Oncology Pharmacy Practice

Designated board-certified oncology pharmacists (BCOP)

Geriatric Pharmacy Practice

Designated certified geriatric pharmacist (CGP)

Additional information can be located on the BPS website at http://www.bpsweb.org/08_Resources.html.

The value of certification is evident on many levels. Box 10.7 lists additional organizations that provide healthcare-focused certification. Although the fundamental intent of certification has been to enhance patient care, current board-certified pharmacists have reported both personal and professional benefits. Board-certified practitioners have reported increased marketability and acceptance by other healthcare professionals, and improved feelings of self-worth, which differentiates them from general practice pharmacists.[19] Some board-certified pharmacists have received financial rewards including salary increase, job promotion, bonus pay, and direct compensation for services. Board certification is a respected and accepted credential that can be listed on credentialing, privileging, and collaborative drug therapy management applications to gain access to advanced practice areas.

Box 10.7 • Additional Organizations Providing Healthcare Focused Certifications

- American Board of Clinical Pharmacology (www.abcp.net) offers a certification exam in clinical pharmacology.
- American Board of Toxicology (www.abtox.org) offers a certification exam in toxicology.
- American Association of Diabetes Educators (www.aadenet.org) offers a certification exam in diabetes education.
- American College of Healthcare Executives (www.ache.org) offers a certification exam in healthcare management.
- National Institute for Standards in Pharmacist Credentialing (www.nispcnet.org) offers certification exams in disease state management, including asthma, diabetes, dyslipidemia, and anticoagulation.

It has been suggested that board certification of clinical pharmacy practitioners should be used as a marker of quality because it is an indicator of an individual's knowledge at a predefined level that has been rigorously validated. Further, board certification should be adopted as an expectation of clinical pharmacy practitioners to meet the JCPP Vision of Pharmacy Practice.[20] To further strengthen the case for board certification, academic recommendations for pharmacists involved in precepting students also urge pharmacy practice faculty to pursue board certification and suggest that faculty with patient care responsibilities be board certified.[21] A more recent report suggested minimum hiring qualifications for clinical faculty should include 2 years of residency training, 3 years' experience in a progressive clinical practice, or board certification.[22] In addition the ASHP Accreditation Standard for pharmacy residency programs requires that when certification is offered in the specialty of your residency a residency program director should be board certified.[23]

• Preceptor Pearls •

If you are a preceptor that works in an organization that may have more than one student at a time, schedule a lunch discussion with the students and include one or two other preceptors. Have the students participate in an informal debate and discussion regarding key career issues such as ambulatory versus hospital practice, rationale for residencies and fellowships, and the importance of obtaining advanced credentials. When moderated effectively by a preceptor, these types of peer interactions can be very enlightening to a student.

Additional Career Planning Support

Once the student has made a well-informed decision regarding a particular career path, there is still much that a preceptor can offer to further assist the student and help them be successful. Assisting them in developing a network of pharmacist contacts is one important element. This can be accomplished in a variety of ways, but one of the easiest is to take them to a local or state professional meeting or continuing education program. Introduce the student to the people you know and encourage them to "work the room" and meet others, with a focus on helping the student connect with pharmacists in their desired career path. Take the student to as many hospital, business, or other types of meetings as possible and make sure that they are welcomed. Introduce them to your supervisor and others in leadership roles. Helping students develop relationships with physicians, nurses, and other healthcare professionals will not only improve their rotation experience, but could also open career path doors later on.

The preceptor can also provide help to the student by reviewing their curriculum vitae (CV) and ensuring that key elements of their experience and education are highlighted and detailed to match their career goals. You may want to share your CV with the student to provide them with another example and format. Many colleges of pharmacy work with students on resume development, and additional review by the preceptor can be very helpful.

Location is another important consideration to discuss with students. Many students find comfort in staying close to home when looking for their first job or residency program and there may be family reasons that limit relocation prospects. On the other had, the point at which they complete their degree is often a period in life where graduating students are most mobile. Where applicable, speak with students about organizations and programs that may be outside of their perceived geographic boundaries. This is especially pertinent for students that want a specific type of residency or specialty opportunity or would like to pursue a career in a more unique practice setting.

Students that have decided on a specific career path should be coached regarding the importance of doing additional research as they identify organizations where they may want to seek employment. Just as they would research information on a major purchase, they should also critically evaluate potential employers. Understanding the organization's patient population, mission, and current financial status can help clarify potential employment choices. If possible, encourage the student to speak with other pharmacists from that company that are in similar positions.

Finally, helping the student polish their interview skills can be very valuable. Develop a set of common interview questions and pose one or two of these questions to the student every week. Role playing answers to specific questions can also prepare the student for the job seeking process. Using common questions like "What are your strengths and weakness?" or "What makes you well-suited for this role?" are good questions to start with. Using behavioral-based questions such as "Tell me about how you would handle a situation where a physician disagreed with you and you knew you were right?" can help prepare the student for some of the tougher interviews that they may experience (see pearl).

• Preceptor Pearls •

Sample open-ended and behavioral interview questions that can help prepare a student for the real thing.

- What tips or tricks do you use to make your job easier or increase your effectiveness?

- You receive a phone call from a nurse that is very angry and rude, saying that she has been waiting five hours for pharmacy to send an antibiotic. What do you do?

- Tell me about an instance where you changed your opinion after receiving new information.

- Describe a work or school situation where your behavior served as a model for others.

- You find out that you have made a medication error. It's minor and likely that no one will ever know. What do you do?

- How do you decide what gets top priority when you schedule your time?

- Tell me about a time when you had to deal with a difficult boss or coworker. Physician?

- What are the most important things that you expect to find at our organization (benefits, salary, job responsibilities, advancement, etc.)?

Summary

Rewarding careers are the result of thoughtful planning, effort, and sacrifice. The preceptor's role is to help students understand the importance of career planning, help them discover their interests and aptitudes for possible careers, and learn more about the available careers for pharmacists. It is also important for preceptors and students to learn the appropriate considerations related to credentialing and that further credentials can be invaluable to a student's future success. The preceptor's potential impact on a student's career is virtually limitless and can result in a professional relationship that spans decades. Being part of a student's career planning efforts is rewarding and may even provide insight into the preceptor's own career path.

References

1.   Giorgianni SJ. *Full Preparation: The Pfizer Guide to Careers in Pharmacy.* New York, NY: Pfizer Pharmaceutical Group; 2001.

2.   Purdue University, School of Pharmacy and Pharmaceutical Sciences. Becoming a pharmacist: career opportunities for pharmacy. Available at: www.pharmacy.purdue.edu/students/prospective/careeropts.php. Accessed September 22, 2008.

3. Academy of Managed Care Pharmacy. The role of pharmacists in managed health care organizations. Available at: www.amcp.org. Accessed September 22, 2008.

4. American Society of Consultant Pharmacists. Available at: www.ascp.com. Accessed September 27, 2008.

5. Murphy JE, Nappi JM, Bosso JA, et al. ACCP Position Statement. American College of Clinical Pharmacy's vision of the future: postgraduate pharmacy residency training as a prerequisite for direct patient care. *Pharmacotherapy.* 2006;26:722–33.

6. Anon. Professional policies approved by the 2007 ASHP House of Delegates. *Am J Health Syst Pharm.* 2007;64:e68–e71.

7. Lee, M, Bennett M, Chase P, et al. Final report and recommendations of the 2002 AACP Task Force on the Role of Colleges and Schools in Residency Training. *Am J Pharm Educ.* 2004;68:1–19.

8. American Society for Health-System Pharmacists. ASHP accreditation standard for postgraduate year one (PGY1) pharmacy residency programs. Available at: http://www.ashp.org/s_ashp/docs/files/ RTP_PGY1AccredStandard.pdf. Accessed October 1, 2008.

9. Teeters JL. New ASHP pharmacy residency accreditation standards. *Am J Health Syst Pharm.* 2006;62:1012–4, 1018.

10. Directory of Residencies, Fellowships, and Graduate Programs. Available at: http://www.accp.com/resandfel/. Accessed October 1, 2008.

11. American Association of Colleges of Pharmacy. Joint Commission of Pharmacy Practitioners (JCPP) vision statement. Available at: http://www.aacp.org/Docs/MainNavigation/Resources/ 8597_JCPPVisionStatement.pdf . Accessed June 23, 2008.

12. Accreditation Council for Pharmacy Education. Accreditation standards and guidelines for the professional program in pharmacy leading to the doctor of pharmacy degree. Available at: http://www.acpe-accredit.org/ pdf/ACPE_Revised_PharmD_Standards_Adopted_Jan152006.pdf. Accessed October 2, 2008.

13. Burke JM, Miller WA, Spencer AP, et al. Clinical pharmacist competencies. *Pharmacotherapy.* 2008;28(6):806–15.

14. National Committee for Quality Assurance. Available at: http://www.ncqa.org/tabid/58/Default.aspx. Accessed October 2, 2008.

15. Galt KA. Credentialing and privileging for pharmacists. *Am J Health Syst Pharm.* 2004;61:661–70.

16. The Council on Credentialing in Pharmacy. Credentialing in pharmacy: The Council on Credentialing in Pharmacy. *Am J Health Syst Pharm.* 2001;58:69–76.

17. The Council on Credentialing in Pharmacy. Credentialing in pharmacy. July 2006. Available at: http:// www.ascp.com/education/certification/upload/CCPWhitePaper2006.pdf. Accessed October 2, 2008.

18. Board of Pharmaceutical Specialists. Available at: http://www.bpsweb.org/Home.html. Accessed September 30, 2008.

19. Pradel FG, Palumbo FB, Flowers L, et al. White paper: value of specialty certification in pharmacy. *J Am. Pharm Assoc.* 2004;44:612–20.

20. Saseen JJ, Grady SE, Hansen LB, et al. Future clinical pharmacy practitioners should be board-certified specialists. *Pharmacotherapy.* 2006;26(12):1816–25.

21. Spinler SA, Boss J, Hak L, et al. Report of the task force concerning board certification requirements for pharmacy practice faculty. *Am J Pharm Ed.* 1997;61:213–6.

22. Lee MI, Bennett M, Chase P, et al. Final report and recommendations of the 2002 AACP task force on the role of colleges and schools in residency training. *Am J Pharm Educ.* 2004;68:article S2.

23. American Society of Health-System Pharmacists. ASHP accreditation standard for postgraduate year two (PGY2) pharmacy residency programs. Available at: http://www.ashp.org/s_ashp/docs/files/ RTP_PGY2AccredStandard.pdf. Accessed June 23, 2008.

Power in organizations is the capacity generated by relationships.
Margaret Wheatly

Our success has really been based on partnerships from the very beginning.
Bill Gates

Chapter 11

Partnerships with Schools

David D. Allen, Louis D. Barone, Cindi Brennan, Todd W. Canada,
Cynthia A. Clegg, Bradi L. Frei, Sarah E. Lake-Wallace, Roland A. Patry,
Michael Piñón, Kevin Purcell, Jennifer L. Ridings-Myhra, Cynthia Wilson

Chapter Outline

Learning Objectives

- Explain why schools of pharmacy and practice sites enter into partnerships.
- Describe two benefits of educational affiliation agreements to each of the following: the preceptor, the school of pharmacy, and the site.
- Explain the process of and reasoning for continuous quality improvement once the experiential education begins.
- Describe how a partnership agreement between a school of pharmacy and an affiliated practice site can enhance preceptor training and development.
- Describe how student support and financial issues can affect the creation of a partnership affiliation between a school of pharmacy and practice site.
- Explain how documenting positive outcomes can affirm the value of the partnership and justify the allocation of additional resources.
- Learn to develop precepting methods to excel as a clinical instructor, an evaluator, a role model and as a mentor.
- Discuss the contents of written educational affiliation agreements.
- Establish a method to attain and enhance precepting skills.
- Recognize and participate in activities that will make you a better preceptor.
- Describe the purpose of providing feedback to the school regarding student preparedness and educational outcomes.
- Describe the importance of expectations.
- Explain the importance of partnering with the school to address difficult or failing students.

Developing Partnerships: The Preceptor Perspective

Importance of a Partnership

Developing a partnership can be beneficial both ways since a facility/institution and the school/college of pharmacy may achieve more as a whole than individually. Examples include having more resources available by sharing associated costs or pooling resources, greater impact in direct patient care with a larger staff including students, and reducing overall costs of care with new and possibly better ways of managing medication usage (e.g., incorporating guidelines). Both parties can learn continually from a partnership with effective communication and support for each other. Generally, the more benefits seen within a partnership strengthen the commitment each individual entity has toward it. Mutual benefits are always observed when working together to care for patients and their families, our staff and students, and the communities served. Partnerships develop leadership, trust, learning, and performance management within each entity, and its overall uniqueness contributes to greater collaboration.

The preceptor's practice site and the school of pharmacy must develop a true partnership in order to ensure success of the experiential education program for everyone involved. Partnership development takes time and effort but is critical to success especially if multiple schools of pharmacy use any one site. Both partners must spend time initially to learn the needs and expectations of one another. It is often necessary to compare the needs and expectations to any existing relationships with other schools of pharmacy. It is also important to understand the operation and culture of both organizations. The chances of building a successful long-term partnership are much greater if the site's practice model and the school's education and training program fit well together, and if the mission, vision, philosophy, and core values of both partners are in alignment.

A partnership may be defined by what is written in the formal educational affiliation agreement, but the success is determined by the relationships developed between key persons at the practice site and at the school of pharmacy. The preceptor or pharmacy director in charge of coordinating the experiential education program at the site and the assistant/associate dean responsible for experiential education or his or her designee at the school need to work closely together and have periodic contact. This relationship is very important as the school administrator will be the site coordinator's primary contact person and interface with the school. Having a good relationship is especially important when trouble-shooting problems and dealing with difficult students. It is also of critical importance when staffing vacancies or emergencies occur within a practice site affecting the feasibility of student rotation schedules.

Establishing the Partnership

A site visit during which the site coordinator and the school administrator can meet will allow them to begin forming their relationship. All preceptors within a site should attend the site visit; they can all benefit from the meeting by getting to know the school administrator and understanding his or her expectations, and vice-versa. Preceptors and school administrators can exchange information about the training opportunities at the site and the experiential education program requirements. The school may request specific documentation of each site preceptor's credentials and training (including preceptor licensure where applicable) prior to providing any type of faculty appointment within the school. Typically, schools will provide rotation-specific experiential education manuals that contain the goals and objectives, required learning activities and assignments, and evaluation form(s). At this point, the practice site coordinator and its preceptors should compare their own internal documents for student rotations to see what additional requirements of their time and resources may be needed. By working closely with the school, preceptors are often able to acquire needed resources that were not previously available at the site. The potential types of rotations and the number of preceptors available should be discussed, as well as the site capacity for students on a monthly and annual basis. The site and the school should agree on the optimal preceptor-to-student ratio for each available rotation and confirm this with their respective State Board of Pharmacy for verification of supervised hours if applicable. This will be important when the site coordinator and school administrator work on constructing a schedule for student placement. Ultimately, a shared vision and plan for the future should be created. Then both site and school can budget for and allocate the necessary resources to accomplish mutual goals and objectives in a structured and timely manner. Future plans could include such things as slowly increasing the number of students per month, developing additional elective rotations, hiring more clinical pharmacists, recruiting and placing a faculty member(s) at the site, and developing or expanding residency programs at the site. Depending on the practice site and preceptor contribution to the school, plans could also be formulated for an on-site preceptor training program or access to online versions of preceptor training modules. This may be the only opportunity some preceptors will have to interact with the school administrator or other preceptors in a given region and especially in remote practice sites.

• Preceptor Pearls •

Establishing and maintaining a good relationship with the school administrator will help solve problems relating to the pharmacy practice experience within the practice site more efficiently.

Although the educational affiliation agreement does not determine the success of the partnership, it is an important legal document as it defines the requirements for each partner. An educational affiliation agreement should be in place before students begin experiential education at a practice site. This can be a time-consuming process, especially if changes to the school's standard educational affiliation agreement are proposed either as a result of negotiation between the site coordinator and the school administrator or through review by the site's attorney. In the latter situation, the school's attorney must then approve the proposed changes. Finally, people in each organization with the power to authorize such a partnership must sign the agreement. Both the practice site and the school will retain a copy for their records. Like any business transaction involving a written contract, do not rely on verbal commitments. For example, if the school has offered to pay the site for precepting services or to provide faculty appointments, textbooks, or library access to preceptors, the agreement should include this information either in the body of the text or in an appendix. This can help prevent any misunderstanding and frustration. The preceptor should also construct a rotation-specific outline of student expectations and responsibilities while at the practice site and/or a student contract for accountability (Figure 11.1).

• Preceptor Pearls •

Check with your site coordinator to ensure the educational affiliation agreement is in place and not simply in process before students arrive at the site.

Name (*print*): _____

Preceptor and Site Expectations

Comments

1. Introduce yourself at all first encounters and greet patients and other healthcare professionals with a smile and/or positive inflection in your voice. Speak effectively (*e.g., not condescending, sarcastic, meek, or overly assertive*).	
2. Guard patient information from disclosure and seek permission to disclose information to other parties (*e.g., family, other healthcare professionals*).	
3. Be professional and respectful at all times. Apply knowledge, experience, and skills to the best of your ability.	
4. Demonstrate effective listening skills (*good eye contact, nonverbal cues*) and the willingness and flexibility to contribute to the well-being of others.	
5. Be well-groomed and dress with clothing that is professional in appearance (*e.g., appropriate to the culture of the institution/facility as defined by the preceptor, site dress code, and professional norms*). Minimize wearing of jewelry in patient care areas.	
6. Arrive each day prepared with equipment and assignments. Demonstrate a sense of duty and earnest desire to learn.	
7. Contact preceptor if you are to be physically absent (*e.g., sick*) from a rotation site. Submission of experiential education hour sheets indicating absences at the rotation site that are not reported to preceptor are subject to disciplinary actions.	
8. Notify preceptor if you must work at a job outside of your rotation for >16 hr/week.	
9. Actively participate in all rotational experiences (*e.g., patient rounds, meetings, discussions, counseling*) and complete all requested assignments on time without plagiarism. Demonstrate accountability without repeated reminders.	
10. Do more than you think you can on your rotational experiences (*e.g., request projects to avoid being idle*).	
11. Maintain your student portfolio and actively share with each student, preceptor, and potential employer.	
12. Be present and actively participate in all requested site meetings and presentations.	
13. Meet all requested site deadlines for submission of assignments and presentations.	
14. Submit complete experiential education paperwork at least 48 hours prior to the end of the rotation.	
15. Provide constructive feedback on each preceptor and site after each rotation (*good or bad*) by the deadline given.	
16. Be present for and pass all required student exams (*clinical, community, institutional*) on the assigned dates.	
17. Actively participate in professional organizations and community service.	
18. Investigate professional career options from preceptors, students and the community.	

I have received training on the above expectations and understand my responsibilities.

_____

Student Signature   Date

Figure 11.1. Sample student contract.

Benefits for Preceptors

As we have discussed in other chapters, the intrinsic rewards of precepting are great. However, because of partnerships with schools, there are also a number of extrinsic rewards. Rewards alone are not necessarily motivation for a pharmacist to become a preceptor, but research concerning the motivators for pharmacy preceptors is deficient; most literature concerning reasons preceptors perform this vital service is based on medical educators. In 2006, as reported in the *Journal of the American Pharmacy Association,* Skrabel et al. found preceptors reported increases in their enjoyment of the practice of medicine (82%); time spent reviewing clinical medicine (66%); desire to keep up with recent developments in medicine (49%); and patients' perception of their stature (44%).[1] Furthermore, these authors reported their own experiences in precepting pharmacy students during their advanced practice experiences citing their expectations during the rotation and approach to teaching students.

In 1999, Kumar et al. reported the most common incentives offered to medical practitioners for assisting medical schools with clinical experiences for their students included appreciation letters, special recognition events, academic appointments, and educational opportunities.[2] It is equally important for schools to consider what opportunities they have to provide recognition, considering the 1995 article by Dr. Zarowitz in which he described pharmacy practitioners as having a "fundamental need to be noticed, to feel important, and to be recognized for excellence."[3] A preceptor who has received multiple Preceptor of the Year awards states that her reason for precepting was that it "allows current pharmacy practitioners to remain up-to-date with medical information. Also, the preceptor's own knowledge of the material improves while teaching it to students." Additional reasons for precepting voiced by pharmacy practitioners include the following: enhancement of the practitioner's knowledge of the subject area as a direct result of student questions; giving back to the profession; and the generating of research hypotheses from some students' questions. For experiential education coordinators, it is important to understand what motivates a pharmacist to be a preceptor in order to determine what benefit will be the most meaningful. The reasons for becoming a preceptor are unique to the individual and are usually multifactorial. The reasons for precepting and its perceived benefits may be divided into two categories, tangible and intangible, and are discussed below.

Tangible benefits include the following:

- Access to drug information. Preceptors should inquire if access to online library resources and library privileges are available, including access to textbooks and journals. Not all colleges are in control of these offerings, but for preceptors who have limited library offerings this can provide an excellent resource.

- Access to free continuing education programs. The efforts to move the profession of pharmacy toward CPD increase the need for specific educational programs. Whether offered specifically for a practice site or as part of school specific program, continuing education programs can be fit into both the needs and goals of all parties.

- Adjunct faculty appointments. The awarding and designation of formal adjunct faculty appointments has been embraced by many pharmacy schools and universities. Furthermore, this practice has been widely adopted by medical schools.[1,2] These titles and awards can be utilized to recognize and honor deserving and dedicated practitioners that have committed their time as preceptors and as mentors to the school's students. In addition to these faculty appointments serving as a reward, they can also serve as an incentive for practitioners to become involved with and committed to the school through establishing new or maintaining existing rotations for students.

- Awards (e.g., Preceptor of the Year). Recognitions of this level are a source of pride for the individual preceptor and his or her practice site. It can also be used for advancement in the profession via salary increases or for earning recognition from pharmacy professional organizations, such as in conferment of fellow status.

- Educational newsletters. Not only do newsletters provide general school information, they can also be used to highlight and recognize activities of preceptors.

- Free access to college specific entertainment events (i.e., football and theatre)

- In-kind gifts. These gifts may vary but receiving a gift bearing the school's name or emblem can be a source of pride for practitioners and give a sense of belonging and community. Common in-kind gifts are a college pocket emblem or a lapel pin for a lab coat.

- Invitation to college events (e.g., White Coat Ceremonies, commencement ceremonies, receptions at national meetings). School events can generate a considerable amount of pride and sense of acceptance among practitioners. Many of these events can bring back fond memories of the milestones one has already reached, as well as provide opportunities to reconnect with former colleagues and instructors.

- Stipend or salary

- Support for professional meetings. This type of benefit may not be readily available from all schools but can be very meaningful to practitioners.

- Support in research, grant writing, drug utilization reviews, and quality and performance improvement projects. Most practitioners realize the importance of quality and performance projects; however, when staffing is tight these areas often do not get the necessary attention. Students can bring a level of energy and experience to these types of activities. In addition, the school can benefit from research opportunities.

- Computer support

• Preceptor Pearls •

Familiarize yourself with the benefits of your site's educational affiliation agreements and take advantage of every opportunity to help you become a better preceptor.

Intangible benefits can include the following:

- Involvement in faculty committees and special projects. Many people seek for a way to give back to their profession. Invitations to participate at this level can provide that opportunity as well as reinforce the level of respect a school has for an individual by requesting input on these activities.

- Networking opportunities with other practitioners. Having a common bond/tie to other practitioners can be very useful when questions arise in your pharmacy practice or while trying to develop new clinical services.

- Certificates. Though a piece of paper may not have financial value, the reminder of the importance and appreciation of the role of the preceptor can be very meaningful. These certificates when posted in general areas can also lead to other individuals recognizing the role the preceptor plays.

- Cognitive. Students provide a different perspective and may ask questions you have never considered. Teaching is an excellent learning tool and improves your own level of expertise in the subject area.

- Recognition. Preceptors appreciate being recognized for their contribution to the education of future pharmacists. Recognition can be achieved through verbal acknowledgement at school events, certificates, awards, written acknowledgment in a preceptor section of school newsletter, and appreciation letters, among other ways.

- Emotional. A thank-you note directly from a student or from the school can convey the simple emotion of gratitude that many individuals appreciate.

- Develop and maintain clinical activities and services for patients. Students can be given the task to help develop a new clinical service, which is both educational and exciting for the student and very important and valuable to the preceptor.

- Help with workload, especially during employee vacations

- Provide more personalized counseling for patients. The progress toward improved patient outcomes has been limited by the ability to change patient behaviors. Additional counseling opportunities, due to increased manpower (i.e., student pharmacists), can help improve the lives of the patients.

- New perspective on existing or new projects. It is easy to get tunnel vision when working in the same facility or project for an extended period of time. The student can benefit the preceptor by asking new questions and by providing a new perspective because he or she does not already see the conclusion at the beginning of the project. Students also bring a variety of experience from their rotations that can provide unique and helpful perspectives. The students have more time than you do, in most cases. You can direct their experience to include a significant amount time to a specific project that gives them a quality learning experience and is beneficial to you.

- Keep abreast of current medications and treatment modalities. Many practitioners quickly learn it is difficult to stay current after leaving the academic setting. Either through teaching the needs of the students, journal club presentation, or general discussions, students and schools can help keep the atmosphere of learning current.

- Participate in the training of future pharmacists

- Give back to the profession

- Participate in the evolution of the profession

There is never one universal answer to what motivates an individual or what is truly valued. "The list of ideas for ways to recognize and reward preceptors is not meant to be exhaustive; implementing some of these ideas along with other creative reward mechanisms can help build camaraderie, unity, communication, and respect between full-time faculty members and preceptors. More importantly, it will make preceptors feel good about themselves and the jobs they are doing."[4] Preceptors should provide feedback concerning their role as a preceptor, whether solicited by the school or not. Schools should actively seek ways to benefit preceptors in consideration of the roles they play in student education. Similarly, preceptors should take a moment to consider the benefits they receive from their activities and recognize the impact precepting has on themselves. Considering the new ACPE standards for early experiential education, the important role preceptors play in all levels of student experience should be appreciated continuously and preceptors should receive benefits that are individualized and have meaningful value.

Maintaining a Partnership

After establishing an experiential education program at a practice site, the process of continuous quality improvement (CQI) must begin. There are always opportunities for improvement and lessons to learn in order to become a better preceptor and build a better experience. The preceptor should develop his or her own pre- and post-assessment tool for each rotation and consider having the student determine his or her learning preferences (e.g., http://www.vark-learn.com/english/index.asp) prior to starting the respective rotation. A student's portfolio is also an excellent starting point to determine what specific learning opportunities the preceptor should provide for each rotation. Obtaining student feedback on the preceptors and the practice site is critical to the CQI process. The school administrator should provide a summary of student evaluations of the site and the preceptors on a regular basis. This may be on an annual or semiannual basis depending on the numbers of students precepted during a given time period. It is important to assure the integrity of the evaluation process and maintain anonymity of comments in order to obtain honest and useful information. Additionally, the preceptor can hold a debriefing session at the end of each rotation and obtain timely oral and/or written feedback from students for the purposes of CQI. Some practice sites have successfully developed and implemented a separate student questionnaire (e.g., Survey Monkey) regarding the specific preceptor and rotation to provide more timely alterations as needed for optimal experiences on both ends.

The school administrator will most likely make periodic site visits. This allows the site coordinator and other preceptors the opportunity to seek his/her advice and for the school administrator to share information on best practices observed in other sites. Preceptors can also tell the school administrator their personal observations regarding student preparedness and assimilation of coursework and experiential competencies. The school administrator may also share the results of formal student testing following experiential training as a component of their milestones in pharmacy education to prepare the students for the North American Pharmacist Licensure Examination.

• Preceptor Pearls •

Take advantage of site visits to discuss best practices at your site and those the school administrator may have observed in other sites.

Preceptors should also actively seek advice and share their ideas, successes, and failures with other preceptors they know. Further, they can share those innovations, success stories, and best practices with their peers by making presentations at preceptor conferences, participating in the American Association of Colleges of Pharmacy's Academic-Practice Partnership Initiative (created in 2004), presenting posters at professional society meetings, and publishing articles in pharmacy journals or other professional preceptor publications.

Positive outcomes may be documented that affirm the value of the partnership and possibly justify the allocation of additional resources. Improvements and desired outcomes may be measured in patient care, education, research, and administrative activities.

Developing Partnerships: The School Perspective

The ACPE accreditation standards for the professional program in schools of pharmacy have been modified to now define experiential education in terms of introductory pharmacy practice experience (IPPE) and advanced pharmacy practice experience (APPE). Introductory experiences (P1-P3) cannot be less than 5% and the advanced experiences (P4) cannot be less than 25% of the curricular length of the professional degree program.[5] There has been considerable discussion within academia regarding the resources and program management requirements to implement the IPPE and APPE programs. It is uncertain if any school of pharmacy would have the resources to meet IPPE and APPE requirements without developing academic partnerships. However, there are many reasons beyond meeting accreditation standards that should be considered when developing partnerships with preceptors including legal, liability, policy and financial concerns.

Benefits to the School

Partnerships evolve because each individual or group perceives a benefit of working together instead of singularly. These benefits should be articulated during the early stages of discussion on forming a partnership for experiential education. The primary benefits for the school include access to a quality practice site for students, increased access to preceptor faculty to participate in didactic teaching, and the opportunity to gain additional recruiting advantage by sharing the partner's contacts or resources.

Some partnership agreements for experiential education may also include provisions for shared salary for clinical faculty based at the facility of the partner. These faculty salary relationships can take numerous forms but one of the most common is that the faculty will be contracted to the partner practice site. In this relationship, the benefit to the practice site is that the practitioners receive the services of an advanced trained practitioner for a reduced cost without accrued liability for retirement, vacation, or healthcare. The school of pharmacy retains the services of a faculty member but shares the cost of that faculty member's salary and benefits with the partner.

These combination faculty support/affiliation arrangements are not without consequences should either party decide to cancel the contract for the experiential training affiliation or the clinical faculty support. Generally, legal counsel or the school business office will provide guidance on whether to bundle educational affiliation agreements and clinical faculty support contracts.

The demand for experiential education partnerships will continue to increase as schools of pharmacy attempt to address the pharmacist manpower shortage by increasing class size and as new schools are established to meet the demand. The increase in partnership agreements has the added benefit of providing more options to students when selecting practice sites for rotations. These affiliations increase opportunities for student learning in specialty practice areas that ordinarily might not be available to the school through its faculty. Software is now available that automates the matching of students with partners and their preceptors based on factors such as availability, educational requirements of the program, or individual training needs.

Preceptor Development from the School Perspective

The development of partnerships for experiential education provides opportunities for the school to engage in preceptor development through traditional orientation programs, continuing education (CE) or continuing professional development (CPD). Schools conduct orientation programs using a variety of formats, ranging from live presentation to streaming video to video tape and usually supplement these presentations with written information in a preceptor manual. If a separate preceptor manual is not used by the school, an alternative is to include a standard section in each rotation manual describing essential elements such as the school's mission, overview of the curriculum and purpose of experiential education, assessment methodologies, and grading philosophies.

Although most schools are still in the very early stages of development of CPD, it offers the opportunity to more formally engage in the development of preceptors as essential members of the academy. ACPE mandates that the school support skills development for both first-timers and other preceptors in such areas as the ability to teach diverse learners.[4]

An essential element of any partnership agreement for experiential education is the on-going evaluation of the site and preceptors by the school. Site evaluation typically takes two forms: periodic quality assurance evaluation of the site to ensure that the program maintains the highest standards of patient care; and preceptor evaluation and feedback that are often a byproduct of student evaluation of the preceptor's ability to provide instruction, engage students as members of the patient care team, or serve as a role model for the profession.

The timeliness of feedback can be a contentious issue between the school and preceptor. The concern from the school's point of view is the potential impact on the assessment and grading process as well as future job opportunities if the preceptor is privileged to individual student evaluation of the site/preceptor. The preceptor's view generally focuses on the inability to address deficiencies in the site or program if timely feedback is not provided. At a minimum, the school should have a policy that defines timely feedback and procedures by which adverse student comments can be addressed with the preceptor or site management in a timely manner. The partnership agreement should also include provisions for addressing a situation where the preceptor believes that the best interests of patient care or site policies and procedures have been compromised or violated.

Maintaining a Partnership

The educational programs of the college work best when integrated with the pharmacy services of their affiliated heath care organizations. Routine visits by school administrators to practice sites can be valuable in helping to build relationships between schools and their preceptors. These interactions allow school representatives to better understand practice site dynamics and issues, heighten awareness and understanding of experiential rotations, and help the preceptors with continuous quality improvement of the experiential education. Student issues regarding their progress, expectations, evaluations, etc., should be addressed at this time. The school should seize every opportunity to establish, maintain, and improve good working relationships with both administrative and clinical staff at these sites.

Preceptors can give feedback to the school on training requirements and student preparation as well as on the school's organization and service provided to them. This is also a great opportunity for the school representatives to provide preceptors with periodic summaries of the students' evaluations of the preceptor and site.

• Preceptor Pearls •

Your honest feedback to the school can help refine the partnership.

Schools should evaluate the performance of preceptors with established criteria, specifically evaluating individuals for the quality and effectiveness of their practice site, and also for the quality of their teaching and mentoring. The evaluation process should consider and acknowledge efforts of preceptor faculty that make contributions toward the advancement of the students' professional development, such as academic and postgraduate advising, career pathway counseling, research, and mentoring activities. Such evaluation criteria should consider not only student evaluations of the preceptor site, but also well-defined objective criteria for professional service, scholarship, and practice success.

Issues with Partnership Agreements: School Perspective

Although the school may develop a very structured experiential program and engage in a thorough discovery and development process for its preceptors, there is no guarantee that the partnership relationship will not suffer problems because of poor communication, lack of commitment to experiential education beyond free labor, or issues of leniency with grades. If the practice site is significantly distant from the school, lack of specificity in the contract about student support can also become an issue.

Many schools of pharmacy have a long-standing tradition of not providing financial remuneration to preceptors or the site for educational services to students. The schools argue that the cost to provide experiential education would exceed budgets if every site required compensation for the time invested by preceptors. Even in situations where the school policies do provide for a small level of compensation to sites or preceptors, some sites will not accept funding. The partnership agreement for experiential education should include within the agreement language or as an attachment, schedule, or exhibit the specific financial considerations involved in the agreement.

The ACPE standards and guidelines mandate the establishment of formal agreements between the school and practice partners. Partnership agreements are built on trust and mutual interests. From the school's perspective, the partnership provides student practice opportunities that might not be available through full-time faculty. From the partner's perspective, the close relationship with a school of pharmacy is an opportunity to advance its practice agenda and impact the educational outcomes of the professional program.

Expectations for the Partnership

Expectations of the preceptor. As with any partnership or agreement between two or more parties, there are expectations and responsibilities involved. The expectations of the preceptor on site can vary, but there are basic administrative and teaching responsibilities that all preceptors must fulfill.

Administrative responsibilities:

- Orient students to the rotation and training site. Clearly identify specific service and personal expectations.

- Introduce to office and ancillary care staff and encourage them to be helpful and make students feel a part of the team.

- Complete a formal written evaluation of student performance during the rotation according to the school's policy.

- Contact the Regional Dean or Experiential Coordinator to discuss issues of concern and student performance.

Teaching responsibilities:

- Serve as a mentor who assists students in applying knowledge and building skills to perform assigned tasks and to problem-solve patient care.

- Provide appropriate training and supervision.

- Challenge students with deliberate and thoughtful questions.

- Allow students to participate in departmental or institutional activities.

- Provide written and verbal feedback to students in a constructive and timely manner.

- Be available, on site, for assistance during assigned tasks, training, and patient care activities.

- Share learning resources (texts, computers, and educational programs) sufficient to increase student knowledge and productivity.

- Assign readings, literature searches, or medical information gathering pertinent to patient care.

- Integrate student's didactic knowledge base into the designated or assigned pharmacy practice site.

Expectations of the student. Experiential education is designed to help students become active participants in providing contemporary pharmacist patient care services. Under the direction of their preceptors, students will integrate their knowledge of pharmacotherapy, disease states, dosage formulations, and pharmacokinetics in developing and assessing therapeutic plans and evaluating drug selection and/or optimization for patients. Each rotation should emphasize outcomes-oriented decision making in clinical situations regarding drug therapy.

Students are expected to attend physician rounds, interprofessional team meetings, attend conferences and discussions, monitor and present assigned patients, and interact with patients and healthcare professionals. Over the course of their experience students will learn to develop recommendations and participate in decisions about drug therapy with regard to efficacy, toxicity, pharmacoeconomics, and unique methods of drug delivery.

At the end of each experiential rotation, students should be able to do the following:

- Dispense and compound prescriptions in accordance with all legal, ethical, and patient care standard practices.

- Prepare sterile and chemotherapeutic products in accordance with the accepted standard of practice.

- Apply case management skills to drug therapy selection, monitoring, and assessment.

- Develop a plan for continuity of care of patients for drug therapy as part of the healthcare team.

- Develop, implement, and document pharmacist patient care plans that manage patient care needs using drug monitoring and physical assessment skills.

- Identify barriers and propose solutions to manage common disease states in traditionally underserved populations with little or no access to the healthcare system.

- Use strategies to improve patient compliance with drug therapy regimens to enhance outcomes.

- Develop practice management skills relating to documentation and compensation issues, managed care, supervision of supportive or technical personnel, and administrative matters related to operations and patient outcomes.

- Demonstrate the ability to integrate distributive and clinical skills in providing pharmacist patient care.

- Actively participate in clinical process improvement activities and population based therapeutic drug decision-making for targeted populations or groups of patients.

- Actively participate in activities related to health promotion and disease prevention in a variety of settings.

In addition, students will maximize their investment in education and the value of their experiential learning program by adhering to these guidelines:

- Contact the preceptor 7 to 10 days prior to the start of the rotation for the schedule, directions to the site, and any other pertinent information.

- Exhibit appropriate professional dress and behavior while on experiential learning assignments.

- Meet deadline established by the experiential learning office, course masters, and preceptors.

- Demonstrate an eagerness to increase knowledge, skills, and abilities through experiential learning.

- Make up any time away from the site for any reason (i.e., illness, religious/school/government holidays, school or personal activities, etc.) during the scheduled rotation dates.

Benefits for Site

It would be difficult for practice facilities to participate in student education and training unless tangible benefits are also apparent to the pharmacy practice facility. Indeed, the labor-intensive activities involved with hosting students on experiential rotations should come with some type of reward. Each site will identify these benefits in ways appropriate to the practice setting, and educational institutions will provide these based on their means.

Defining the Role of Pharmacists

In limited resource pharmacy sites where the college provides faculty preceptors, the role of pharmacists can often be elevated to include patient-centered and evidence-based care, instead of only distributive and minimal clinical services. This could lead to formal and informal medication consultations, patient care rounds, and more committee involvement, while hopefully not negatively impacting the overall pharmacy workload, as the contribution of the college faculty to patient care drives pharmacy services to the forefront. Students on advanced experiential rotations could also assist with medication reconciliation, drug information, discharge counseling, and reporting of adverse medication events.[6] Their cost-effective involvement could lead to improved patient care and safety. Communications between the college and the practice site can improve with specific information exchanged addressing student performance (similar to employees within the practice site), academic and professional misconduct, and harassment and discrimination policies for preceptors and students.

Financial and Resource Implications

Benefits can be monetary, in kind, or nonmonetary. Monetary remuneration, in the form of payment for student rotations, or partial or full salary for cofunded pharmacist staff/faculty preceptors, is a type of arrangement that can be made between the practice facility and the educational institution. In-kind benefits can include access by the facility to university resources not otherwise available, such as online libraries and databases, or access of the site to software, computers, reference books, educational programming, and other resources at reduced or no cost.

Students can demonstrate their value to a practice site from a variety of methods including those pertinent to regulatory agencies, such as The Joint Commission. They can monitor and document pharmacist patient care including medication reconciliation, provide adverse drug event monitoring, perform drug usage evaluations, deliver patient education, present therapeutic alternatives (e.g., formulary cost savings), and reduce drug expenditures.[1,6,7]

• Preceptor Pearls •

Take advantage of the site benefits of the partnership, in addition to your own benefits as a preceptor.

Educational and Competence Implications

The informational resources from the college combined with the faculty's teaching skills contribute to continuing professional development for pharmacists and other healthcare professionals within the practice site. Students also contribute to practice site learning by providing written drug information (often circulated within the pharmacy via a monthly newsletter), in-service presentations, and patient case presentations. The development of practice site competence comes from continual learning and the enhancement of critical thinking and problem-solving skills through practice, as provided by the college faculty and students.[8]

Another benefit can be the development of preceptor training for the practice site by meaningful instruction from the college. The American Association of Colleges of Pharmacy (AACP) has developed standards for exemplary pharmacy practice sites and preceptors to include preceptor and student responsibilities. AACP is also in the process of developing a curriculum for preceptor guidance.[9]

Personal and Professional Advancement Implications

Pharmacy administrators often define the nonmonetary, sometimes intrinsic, benefits to the practice site. A select group of pharmacy administrators questioned on this topic has provided the following perspectives on the advantages of participating in pharmacy student education:

- Assists in recruiting future pharmacist employees. In geographic areas of critical shortage, this is described as one of the top advantages to hosting students.
- Shortens training time for possible future employees
- Contributes to the educational mission of the facility
- Increases pharmacy visibility/presence in patient care areas of the facility
- Provides professional development of staff preceptors
- Exposes students to the concept of advanced training within the practice site as post-graduate year 1 and 2 residencies or fellowships
- Helps to maintain relationships with educational institutions in areas outside of the experiential education, such as research
- Allows collaboration with colleges for professional advancement through research endeavors and grant submission

- Supplies creativity to rethink current pharmacy models and responsibilities
- Gains personal satisfaction by serving as teachers and mentors to future pharmacists
- Students are a good resource for special projects to which pharmacy staff can devote little time, and similarly they often help distribute the workload of an individual preceptor so he/she can do more when students are present in the facility
- Students help keep pharmacy staff current in asking questions and students prompt institutions to review practices that may need updating

Therefore, within the array of tangible and intangible advantages described above, it should be possible to determine benefits to the site that either the facility can recognize on its own, and/or that can be provided by the college or school of pharmacy.

• Preceptor Pearls •

Remember that there are more benefits to precepting than just those listed in the formal partnership agreement. Other benefits come from working directly with the students.

Educational Affiliation Agreements

Partnership or educational affiliation agreements for experiential programs have been in existence in some form since the early beginnings of Pharm.D. education. Educational affiliation agreements formalize the relationships between schools and practice sites to provide additional teaching and training resources beyond school-based faculty. They describe in detail the responsibilities of both the facility and the educational institution.

This agreement may originate with either party. If the college or school of pharmacy initiates an agreement and is part of a larger university or system of universities, the affiliation agreement may be standard for all healthcare-related schools, and then defined for each individual program (i.e., pharmacy) in an amendment to the original educational affiliation. In the case where a site originates the affiliation agreement, it could be a standard agreement based with the facility's parent company or owner or it could be specific for the individual institution.

• Preceptor Pearls •

Although you may not be involved in the creation of the educational affiliation agreement, familiarize yourself with it for your day-to-day responsibilities as a preceptor, and provide feedback to your site coordinator and/or the school administrator; your input could help improve the partnership.

The Accreditation Council for Pharmacy Education (ACPE) through its accreditation standards for the Pharm.D. program mandate that schools or colleges of pharmacy develop relationships "within and outside the university" that enhance the mission and goals of the program. Guideline 6.3 of the accreditation standards dictates that agreements

- are formal in that they are signed by representatives of the parties to the agreement;
- define the nature and scope of the affiliation;
- define the legal liability of the parties to the agreement;
- define the financial arrangements between the parties of the agreement; and
- contain terms within the agreement that allow for periodic review.[10]

Guideline 28.2 mandates written agreements with practice sites used for required practice experiences or frequently used elective experiences. It also provides guidance on agreement language such as terms for termination of the agreement; and how to address student support issues such as immunization policies, health services, and malpractice insurance, among others.[11]

Standard areas of responsibility that these agreements usually address include the following[12]:

- Complete identification of both the educational facility and the practice site (full name, location, type of practice, affiliated institutions, etc.)
- Reference to the need for any additional amending agreements
- Method(s) of conflict resolution
- Responsibilities of the facility, including but not limited to the following:
  1. Compliance with all applicable state, federal, and municipal laws, rules and regulations, and with all applicable requirements of accreditation authorities
  2. Permission for a designated university representative to inspect the facilities for the purpose of the educational experience
  3. Appropriate supervision of students by a qualified practitioner and that practitioner's appointment or other recognition within the university (volunteer or adjunct), or articulation of the appointment of the school's faculty to the facility for the purpose of student supervision
  4. Designating a liaison from the facility to the college or school of pharmacy
  5. Providing appropriate space for student activities
  6. Providing equipment, supplies, qualified personnel, and supervised access to patients required for educational activities
  7. Maintaining of all required licenses
  8. Providing an orientation to the facility
  9. Assuming sole responsibility for patient care
- Responsibilities of the educational institution, including but not limited to the following:
  1. Providing the facility with names of the students assigned to the facility
  2. Assigning to the facility only those students who have completed the prerequisites for participation
  3. Designating a university liaison to the facility

4. Developing criteria for student evaluation and grading

5. Requiring students to be covered by professional liability insurance

6. Ensuring that students have complied with all necessary immunizations and medical releases

7. Removing a student from the facility when the student has engaged in professional misconduct as defined within the agreement (e.g., student compromises patient safety or discloses confidential patient information) or has compromised patient care

8. Compliance with accreditation standards

9. Periodic review of the program

10. Ensuring that students are registered, if appropriate, under state law, as interns

11. Ensuring that students have complied with any criminal history checks and drug screens required by the facility

- Terms and termination of agreement and effective date
- Indemnification of either party
- General provisions, including but not limited to the following:

  1. Statement that students in the pharmacy program are not employees of the facility

  2. Student responsibility for transportation and meals

  3. Nondiscrimination clause

  4. Privacy statement(s)

Language that requires the educational institution to guarantee good student mental and physical health is controversial with many universities because of student privacy and disability issues. Additionally, educational institutions cannot guarantee that students will behave professionally or be highly motivated; however, it is imperative to articulate in writing the sequence of events within both the site and the school that are necessitated by unprofessional conduct. The same student privacy laws that protect certain student information (Family Educational Rights and Privacy Act of 1974, or FERPA, is one such regulation) also may, based on legal interpretation on a particular campus, affect the campus policies on student background checks and drug screens.

In addition to these items, agreement regarding payment to the facility or preceptor for student rotations may be included. Alternatively, this can be handled through other types of contracts.

Agreements initiated by the school may also define for the site, at a minimum, the expectations for handling behavior issues, how to conduct learning activities, and how to counsel students that are not meeting expectations. As a baseline, the practice partner should be expected to complete student evaluation forms within the time prescribed by the school; to deliver the instruction as defined in either orientation provided by the school or as described in a rotation manual, and to participate in program planning activities.

The process of establishing and maintaining affiliation agreements can be cumbersome for both the healthcare facility and the educational program. Corporations, facilities, and/or universities need to include language in all formal written agreements that works, to the extent possible, to avoid litigation from other parties. Adding complexity to this is the fact that various groups and/or individuals and/or departments within the facility or university may be involved in the review of contracts. All of these combined factors result in agreements that take months to even years to finalize between contractual parties. This can ultimately delay the assignment of students to a facility. It is incumbent on both parties to search for mechanisms to facilitate this process to the extent possible.

Partnerships are voluntary agreements based on trust that each partner will fulfill the roles that the agreement defines. A successful partnership is more than a contractual agreement—it requires that both partners feel that their interests are equally represented.

Ways to Become a Better Preceptor

An excellent opportunity for nurturing a successful partnership exists between schools of pharmacy and clerkship preceptors. Schools provide critical support and training to preceptors in order maximize the experiential component for students. Precepting is an iterative process that enhances clinical and teaching skills for the preceptor who is fully committed to self-improvement and takes full advantage of school sponsored training. Unlike classroom teaching, the one-on-one preceptor-student relationship demands that the preceptor, tailor the teaching method to meet the student's needs. This individualization allows the acquisition of new skills and builds confidence for the preceptor.

Preparation. The didactic information provided to pharmacy students by school-based faculty comes to life in clinical settings under the guidance of strong preceptors. The Accreditation Council for Pharmacy Education (ACPE) requires schools of pharmacy to provide preceptor training for their preceptor colleagues.[13] It is important to take full advantage of the training sessions provided by professional educators who offer excellent teaching tips and techniques. Be willing and prepared to share precepting challenges and success stories during these sessions, to contribute to the collective group learning process and individual goals of improving precepting skills.

Ideally, contact the student prior to their experiential education start date to prepare each of you for the most successful outcome. The partnership between the preceptor and the student is critical to the student's achievement. Important questions to ask include the following:

- What are the student's professional goals and objectives?
- How much and what type of previous experience has he or she had?
- What did the student like and dislike about previous experiences?
- How best does the student learn (reading, observing, doing, teaching)?
- Why did the student choose your clinical rotation (if he or she had a choice)?
- What are the student's goals and objectives for the clinical rotation?
- What does the student expect from you during the rotation?

The student needs to know where and when to meet you on the first day, but also what to expect during the experiential rotation with you. While understanding expectations is important for the student, it is essential for the preceptor to understand what the student needs as well. Starting off on the right foot will pave the way for open communication throughout the experiential rotation and will provide both the necessary feedback needed to create a valuable learning experience for the student and to improve your own skills.

Getting started. From the beginning of the rotation, provide daily feedback on the student's progress. Cite specific successes each day and offer coaching in areas that need improvement. It is helpful to role-play with the student to practice communicating clinical recommendations before meeting with other healthcare providers, especially if it is early in the rotation experience.

Use these opportunities to fine-tune your own teaching skills. Remind the student that it is a symbiotic relationship and a trusted partnership in which they have the responsibility to provide specific feedback on your role as their mentor. Ask the student if you are meeting the specific educational needs and whether there are any specific suggestions for improving your precepting.

Be patient and persistent. Some students are not comfortable initially being direct with preceptors but will gain confidence over time. Constructive feedback is the greatest gift students can give to you. Creating an environment in which the student feels comfortable providing feedback to the preceptor is critical to obtaining the information needed in order to improve your precepting skills. Utilize active listening techniques and ask clarifying questions.

Evaluation. Regardless of the school of pharmacy's evaluation schedule, take the time to provide the student with a formal progress evaluation each week. This provides opportunity for the student to alter his or her participation to meet expectations and reduces your frustration with under-performing students. During this evaluation, set aside time for the student to evaluate you. Together, you can plan improvements for each of you to sustain a positive rotation experience.

Formal evaluation requires time and thoughtful preparation. Keep track of specific examples you can use to illustrate both achievements and challenges for your student. Ask the student to discuss your achievements and challenges as his or her preceptor. Specifically inquire about his or her favorite and least favorite parts of the rotation and listen carefully to discover hints about your skills as a preceptor.

Finally, make sure you receive feedback through the school of pharmacy's formal evaluation process. Although academic institutions rules vary, most preceptors receive some type of evaluation that can be very useful in self-improvement activities. Ideally, organizations and preceptors should partner with the schools to create the most useful evaluation and feedback tool for students, preceptors and the school. This collaboration leads to continuous improvement for the clerkship programs and preceptors. Evaluations generally focus on the following:

- The preceptor's preparation for the student
- The preceptor's accessibility and willingness to answer questions
- The preceptor's attitude toward the student and toward the clinical experience
- The quality and quantity of feedback
- The independence granted to the student
- The preceptor's ability as a role model

Preceptors and schools of pharmacy rely on each other's unique contributions to produce the highest quality pharmacist graduates. Nurturing this partnership assures that students receive a balanced education that integrates didactics with practice. The additional professional benefit from precepting pharmacy students is the opportunity to "pay it forward." In turn, students will keep you on your toes and encourage your development as a better pharmacist and preceptor by providing challenges. Building your precepting skills assures that your students are well prepared to meet the professional demands they will face and assures a bright future for the profession of pharmacy.

Providing Feedback to Schools to Improve Student Competencies

There is nothing unique about the important elements of a good working relationship with a school. Like in most relationships, good communication and clear expectations are critical. Other chapters discuss the ways of developing effective communication and effective evaluations. Hopefully you, as the preceptor, will be giving only positive feedback to the school, but it is just as important to be honest about problems and issues. There is an important element preceptors bring to the student evaluation process; you have the opportunity to observe their abilities and skills on a one-on-one basis. This is not always possible during didactic learning settings.

Establishing Relationships with Schools

The first step in this process is to establish the appropriate contacts and the best methods for communicating with those individuals. There are several ways to identify who these individuals might be. Consider asking other preceptors who are their contacts, or if you are new to an area check the school websites and send an inquiry e-mail to site coordinators. In developing the initial relationship with the school, ask who is responsible for scheduling the students and who handles performance issues. Contact these individuals before there are any issues in order to help establish a relationship that can be useful in problem solving.

Another important area is to keep up with the required paperwork (evaluations, timesheets, etc.). Schools are usually required to maintain these basic forms to meet accreditation and regulatory standards. By keeping up your end of the responsibility, you can establish a common ground of respect.

Beyond just the direct feedback to the school about performance, feedback on scheduling is important. School coordinators must work with many different sites to coordinate schedules for often hundreds of different students at one time. Help schools plan their schedules by advising them of the dates you will not be available at your work site. It is useful for the school to know if the student is going to have to be in different locations due to a preceptor's vacation or other scheduling conflict. This information allows the school to relocate the student if needed. As soon as you are aware of workflow or staffing changes that will affect your site's ability to take students, you should let the school know. Schedules do change, but advance notice allows the school to find alternative sites or adjust times. If you change your work site, inform the school of this as well. Developing a good relationship with quality preceptors can be difficult. Many schools want to maintain the relationship not only with the site, but also with the individual. The relationship between school and preceptor is important, but for it to be an effective relationship, you must keep an open line of communication.[13]

• Preceptor Pearls •

Be proactive; communicate your needs to the school and ensure you submit any necessary paperwork on time.

Establishing Expectations of the School

At the same time you establish your relationships, you should establish your expectations of the school. Tell them how far in advance you need a schedule of students. Let them know if your site requires any specific paperwork to be completed before students arrive on site. Let them know if there are times that you are not able to take students due to vacations or workload. Tell them the best way to contact you.

In establishing your expectations with the school, ask whether you will be getting student feedback on your activities as a preceptor, and how you will receive that feedback. The school must work to balance the need for honest feedback from the student with the need for preceptor feedback, taking into account the student perceptions of possible negative repercussions if providing critical comments. It is, however, appropriate to ask how and if this feedback might be available.

The school should provide basic goals for rotations. You can use these as a baseline for creating your expectations of the students. Communicate these to the students and use them as a basis of your evaluation. By establishing your expectations with the students, it may help avoid misunderstandings and give them specific goals to work toward. If you find that the goals for a specific rotation need updating or improvement, communicate that with the school as well. This allows for improving future rotations. Remember that, because you work one-on-one with the students, if problems arise, you should also share your expectations with the school so they can understand your point of reference.

• Preceptor Pearls •

It is critical to establish expectations with the students, but it will also benefit the partnership if you communicate your expectations to the school as well.

Sharing Evaluations

The next level of communication should include honest evaluations about student performance. You should try to be as objective as possible and try to limit the influence of personality differences. It can be helpful to review the specific goals of the rotation and relate comments back to these. Likert scales on student skills may be an efficient manner of evaluation, but written comments make it possible to develop a full picture of strengths and weaknesses. Written comments not only improve student understanding of strengths, but also help the school compare activities and skills between rotations.

As with most effective relationships, the communication between schools and preceptors should start early and occur often. If you are having problems with a student, notify the appropriate individuals as early in the rotation as possible. If, in the first weeks of a rotation, a student is not meeting expectations, express your concerns to the school no later than the midpoint of the rotation. This allows time to address specific problems and create a plan to improve the student's outcome. If a student cannot eventually make up the difference, and it is necessary to give a failing grade, the school is now also prepared to make additional plans. Informing the school of the problems you experience with a student allows the school to put together the entire picture if the student protests the grade.

If a student is having difficulty in the experience, consider the following issues:

- Is there a problem integrating knowledge with clinical decisions?
- Is it a communication problem?
- Is there difficulty working effectively with physicians, nurses, or other healthcare providers?

These issues can be difficult to overcome, but it is essential for schools to know about these crucial skills. If a student is having problems with these issues with you as a preceptor, these same problems may continue on other rotations if they are not addressed.

• Preceptor Pearls •

Be sure to address problems as they arise, and communicate them to the school as appropriate.

Working with Problem Students

Preceptors and schools should always undertake all efforts possible to identify any barriers to student success. The first step is, of course, to discuss these issues with students while keeping the school aware of your concerns. The next step is to get the school involved in problem solving. When working with a student who does not meet the minimum requirement, work with the school to develop a plan for improvement. This plan could include moving the student off site until issues can be resolved, assigning additional reading, or providing additional time on a rotation.[14] If these interventions still do not allow the student to progress, and failing the student is necessary, document the actions you took to help the student. The school also needs specific details on how the student failed to meet expectations because the student can appeal that decision. The school cannot accurately represent its side without details. Documentation of all details is important, including concerns about work problems, such as tardiness.

When examining the barriers to success, consider personality issues, cultural issues, personal issues, and lack of knowledge. These problems can make for a difficult preceptor-student relationship, but by specifically addressing them, it may be possible for the student to succeed in the experience. Schools often have experience resolving these issues and can serve as a resource for preceptors as well as a resource for students to find outside help if that is needed.

Issues such as personality differences or cultural influences may not be able to be resolved, but a working relationship is still possible. Though it would be nice to be friends with your student, your primary goal and responsibility is to facilitate learning. Let the school know if you need help addressing these issues or finding ways to create workable solutions.

• Preceptor Pearls •

Before involving the school in problems you have with a student, try to resolve it on your own, while keeping the school informed of the situation.

Failing Students

The school is using you to help teach their students, but it is unreasonable to expect them to have a solution to make each student perform exactly the same way, or to assume the school can solve all problems. Difficult students cannot always be moved from the site. School faculty struggle with how to motivate students just as preceptors do. The schools should be viewed and treated as a partner in developing students into practitioners.

You also should not assume that the school will take care of a problem you do not want to address. If you do not fairly evaluate a student because you do not want to deal with the emotional side of failing a student, the school has no grounds on which to fail a student. Failing a student is hopefully a rare event, but you should always consider the impact the student will have on the profession and future patients. The decision to fail a student should not be taken lightly and will never be an easy experience. Failing a student may ultimately give that person the opportunity to become a better practitioner. Remember, if the student does not meet expectations, it is the student who caused the failure, not you. This relates back to the importance of establishing your expectations early and using these as the focus of your evaluation.

• Preceptor Pearls •

Do not be afraid to fail a student; you just might do him or her a favor. Be sure to fully document your reasons, however, so as to ensure you do not act unjustifiably.

Make sure to document all steps you take to address deficiencies. Let the school know you are intending to fail a student and provide them with documentation as a basis for your decision. Explain to the student how you reached this decision and how he or she can avoid it in the future.[15]

Assimilation of Learning: From Classroom to Patient Room

Finally, if a student has knowledge deficits, it may be possible to assign additional readings or tutorial time. Consider requesting the student to review his or her school notes with you so you can draw parallels from the learning experiences. If you have discovered a significant knowledge deficit that affects a student's performance, the school may have resources to help address the problems as well.[15]

There are many theories on effective teaching styles. Within healthcare education, colleges are moving away from what is known as passive learning (a professor who serves in the role of expert verbalizing information to the learner or student) to more active styles of small group and problem solving styles.[16] However, when the student's reasoning and decisions are going to directly affect a person, the impact on the learner can be significantly different. It is important to emphasize problem solving rather than memorization and discuss the differences in clinical decisions. It is also important to discuss why guessing, even correctly, can result in unnecessary risk to the patient. If the student recommends an unusual or nontraditional treatment plan or does not fully understand the reasoning behind his or her choice, suggest that he or she present evidence from the literature to support the plan. Discuss why it is inappropriate to defend a treatment option with such unsupported statements as, "They say," or "That's what my professor told us." This emphasizes the importance of evidence-based medicine and develops the habit of lifelong learning.

Summary

The job of precepting can be equally rewarding and challenging, but remember that there are resources and tools available. Preceptors should work to access and utilize the tools the schools of pharmacy offer and view them as partners in the student learning experience. Experiential training is just as essential as all other formalized training pharmacy students complete. Colleges of pharmacy work toward improving didactic teaching techniques and experiences, but this is only one step in the process. They also try to find the best instructors for the experiential year—the preceptors. Preceptors help turn classroom learning into hands-on skills. As such, the schools depend on the preceptors to provide truthful evaluations of student skills and judge their ability to be pharmacy practitioners. Preceptors have the unique opportunity to work one-on-one with students and thoroughly evaluate their skills. The schools are dependent on preceptors to share this information.

References

1. Skrabal MZ, Kahaleh AA, Nemire RE, et al. Preceptors' perspectives on benefits of precepting student pharmacists to students, preceptors, and the profession. *J Am Pharm Assoc.* 2006;46(5):605–12.

2. Kumar A, Loomba D, Rohit BS, et al. Rewards and incentives for nonsalaried clinical faculty who teach medical students. *J Gen Intern Med.* 1999;14:370–2.

3. Zarowitz B. Rewards and advancements for clinical pharmacy practitioners. *Pharmacotherapy.* 1995;15(1):99–105.

4. American Council on Professional Education. Accreditation standards and guidelines for the professional program in pharmacy leading to the doctor of pharmacy degree. Standard no. 26, guideline 26.1: college or school and other administrative relationships. Available at: http://www.acpe-accredit.org/standards/default.asp. Accessed April 1, 2008.

5. American Council on Professional Education. Accreditation standards and guidelines for the Professional Program in Pharmacy Leading to the doctor of Pharmacy Degree. Standard No. 10: Curricular Development, Delivery, and Improvement. Available at http://www.acpe-accredit.org/standards/default.asp. Accessed February 16, 2009.

6. Bock LM, Duong M, Williams JS. Enhancing clinical services by using pharmacy students during advanced experiential rotations. *Am J Health Syst Pharm.* 2008:65:566–9.

7. Chase P. Rethinking experiential education (or does anyone want a pharmacy student?). *Am J Pharm Educ.* 2007;71:1–2.

8. American College of Clinical Pharmacy. Clinical pharmacist competencies. *Pharmacotherapy.* 2008;28:806–15.

9. Talley CR. Experiential rotations for pharmacy students. *Am J Health Syst Pharm.* 2006;63:1029.

10. American Council on Professional Education. Accreditation standards and guidelines for the professional program in pharmacy leading to the doctor of pharmacy degree. Standard no. 6, guideline 6.3: college or school and other administrative relationships. Available at: http://www.acpe-accredit.org/standards/default.asp. Accessed April 1, 2008.

11. American Council on Professional Education. Accreditation standards and guidelines for the professional program in pharmacy leading to the doctor of pharmacy degree. Standard no. 28, guideline 28.2: college or school and other administrative relationships. Available at: http://www.acpe-accredit.org/standards/default.asp. Accessed April 1, 2008.

12. Accreditation Standards and Guidelines for the Professional Program in Pharmacy Leading to the Doctor of Pharmacy Degree. Accreditation Council for Pharmacy Education. July 1, 2007. Available at: http://www.acpe-accredit.org/pdf/ACPE_Revised_PharmD_Standards_Adopted_Jan152006.pdf.

13. Woo M. [e-mail]. University of Houston, College of Pharmacy; June 9, 2004.

14. Sayer M, Chaput De Saintonge M, Evans D, et al. Support for students with academic difficulties. *Med Educ.* 2002;36(7):643–50.

15. Kleffner JH, Hendrickson WD. Effective clinical teaching. December 2001. Available at: http://www.utexas.edu/pharmacy/general/experiential/practitioner/edopps.html. Accessed July 7, 2008.

16. Chadwick SM, Bearn DR. Teaching and learning: an update for the orthodontist. *J Orthod.* 2002;29(2):162–7.

Index